THE MACROBIOTIC APPROACH TO CANCER

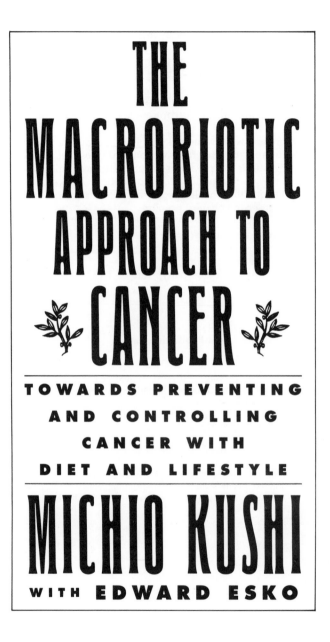

THE MACROBIOTIC APPROACH TO CANCER

TOWARDS PREVENTING AND CONTROLLING CANCER WITH DIET AND LIFESTYLE

MICHIO KUSHI

WITH EDWARD ESKO

AVERY PUBLISHING GROUP INC.

Garden City Park, New York

The medical and health procedures in this book are based on the training, personal experiences and research of the authors. Because each person and situation is unique, the editor and publisher urge the reader to check with a qualified health professional before using any procedure where there is any question as to its appropriateness.

The publisher does not advocate the use of any particular diet and exercise program, but believes the information presented in this book should be available to the public.

Because there is always some risk involved, the author and publisher are not responsible for any adverse effects or consequences resulting from the use of any of the suggestions, preparations, or procedures in this book. Please do not use the book if you are unwilling to assume the risk. Feel free to consult a physician or other qualified health professional. It is a sign of wisdom, not cowardice, to seek a second or third opinion.

Cover design by Abby Kagan
Cover photo by Greg Goebel
In-house editor: Linda Comac
Typesetting by Straight Creek Company, Denver, CO

Library of Congress Cataloging-in-Publication Data

Kushi, Michio.
  The macrobiotic approach to cancer : toward preventing and
controlling cancer with diet and lifestyle / Michio Kushi with Ed.
Esko.
    p. cm.
  Includes bibliographical references and index.
  ISBN 0-898529-486-9
  1. Cancer—Prevention. 2. Cancer—Nutritional aspects.
3. Macrobiotic diet. I. Esko, Edward. II. Title.
  [DNLM: 1. Diet, Macrobiotic—popular works. 2. Life Style-
-popular works. 3. Neoplasms—diet therapy—popular works.
4. Neoplasms—prevention and control—popular works. QZ 201 K97m]
RC268.K89 1991
616.99′405—dc20
DNLM/DLC
for Library of Congress   91-18034
                                                     CIP

Printed in the United States of America

10 9 8 7 6 5 4 3 2 1

Contents

For those of us suffering from an "incurable" disease, for which orthodox medicine offers no remedy, the biggest single benefit that macrobiotics can offer is hope. That was the message that Michio gave me four years ago—that our bodies can reject the illness, that we ourselves are back in charge. We are no longer passively relying solely on doctors, drugs, and hospitals.

In all his writing and lectures, Michio has never forgotten that personal salvation is not enough. He has never ceased to speak of peace and the environment. While we and our children embark on a healthier way of life, we cannot afford to ignore the millions of men and women who are starving. As we ourselves seek to eat fresh and wholesome uncontaminated food, we cannot afford to forget that worldwide commercial empires are still being built on pesticides and artificial fertilizers, on the chemical doctoring of most of the foodstuff in our shops and supermarkets.

If our aim is truly "One Peaceful World," we cannot forget that vast industries are still engaged in the enormously profitable business of producing ever-more lethal weapons of war, that governments pleading poverty can still find astronomical sums to spend on war and destruction. Yet times are changing. By deciding to make ecology the theme of our next International Macrobiotic Congress in Europe, we have shown that we are well aware of this.

Those of us who have come to macrobiotics have an immense responsibility to give leadership to the things we believe in, to work with all men and women of good will to build a new society, freed from ruthless exploitation of man and nature for commercial gain—to build "One Peaceful World." This is what macrobiotics means to me—and I believe this is the message that others will find in this book.

Hugh Faulkner, M.D.
Chianti
Italy

THE MACROBIOTIC APPROACH TO CANCER

Introduction

In many ways, cancer is a symbol of the destructive trends that confront us all in the final decade of the twentieth century. The crisis in personal and global health, in which cancer plays a major role, is rapidly approaching a critical stage, and may soon threaten the continuation of society. In order to reverse this destructive trend and avert future catastrophe, we need to change our way of thinking and look beyond partial or symptomatic answers. If, through self-reflection, we are able to discover the most basic, universal principles that govern the natural world and use them to secure a healthy and peaceful way of life, we will have discovered a fundamental solution to the modern crisis.

Central to this new understanding is a respect for the importance of diet. Throughout the world, cancer, heart disease, and other chronic illnesses have increased in incidence as people shifted from their more balanced traditional dietary patterns. Diets that had been based around whole grains, organically grown fresh vegetables and fruits, beans and sea vegetables, and other regional products, were replaced by a diet based on increased consumption of meat and dairy products, fatty and oily foods, and refined or synthetic food items. Simply put, the rise of cancer and other chronic illnesses is due primarily to the changing dietary habits of modern civilization.

Among the endless varieties of disease, two apparently opposite categories of causes and symptoms stand out. Some circulatory disorders involve overexpansion of the heart and blood vessels, leading to low blood pressure; in other such disorders, the circulatory vessels are overly contracted, leading to high blood pressure. Similarly, there are two apparently opposite categories of cancer; those that appear toward the periphery of the body, such as skin or breast cancer, and those that appear in the internal organs and depths of the body, such as colon, liver, or pancreatic cancer. Regardless of its symptoms, cancer in all of its manifestations can be understood in terms of these opposite tendencies, which, in macrobiotics, are known as yin and yang.

The solution to cancer and other chronic illnesses lies ultimately in eating so that these opposite tendencies are brought into moderate balance. Because we are able to exercise control over what we eat and drink, food is the most important factor influencing the health and happiness of individuals and society. Our ability to control other environmental factors is limited in comparison to the freedom that we exercise when selecting daily foods. Control over daily dietary practice is, therefore, essential in solving the problems of personal and planetary health. The standard macrobiotic diet presented in this book is based on balancing opposites and is similar to diets that kept people in traditional cultures free of cancer. A naturally balanced diet, adapted for personal needs, is the cornerstone of the macrobiotic approach, as are appropriate physical activity and positive mental outlook.

Over the past thirty years, thousands of people in all corners of the globe have recovered from cancer and other chronic illnesses through the macrobiotic approach to diet and way of life. Their stories have been told in lectures and seminars around the world, in newspaper and magazine articles, on radio and television, and in books (e.g., *Healing Miracles from Macrobiotics* by Jean and Mary Alice Kohler; *Recalled By Life* by Anthony Sattilaro, M.D., and Tom Monte; *Macrobiotic Miracle: How a Vermont Family Overcame Cancer* by Virginia Brown and Susan Stayman; *Recovery: From Cancer to Health through Macrobiotics* by Elaine Nussbaum;

Confessions of a Kamikaze Cowboy by Dirk Benedict; *Beating the Odds* by Hugh Faulkner, M.D.; and *Cancer-Free: Profiles of People Who Recovered from Cancer Naturally* by Anne Fawcett and the East West Foundation). As these and other experiences demonstrate, the recovery of physical health often leads to a subtle but profound change in one's entire personality, including the development of more satisfying personal relationships and a deep appreciation for life on all levels. It is through positive changes such as these that a peaceful solidarity can develop within society, leading to the establishment of a peaceful world community.

The Macrobiotic Approach to Cancer is compiled from my articles and lectures over the past seventeen years. It is based on an earlier book—one of the first on macrobiotics and cancer—published in 1981. In this new, revised edition, we introduce the principles of macrobiotics and apply them to the problem of cancer. Also included are personal accounts of exceptional patients who, in spite of the odds, adopted the macrobiotic diet and lifestyle and recovered their health. A review of current cancer and diet research, and guidelines issued by public health agencies that point to the role of a naturally balanced diet in cancer prevention are presented as well. This basic, introductory book offers a general overview of the macrobiotic approach and complements the more extensive presentation featured in *The Cancer Prevention Diet* (St. Martin's Press, 1983), my other major book on the topic of cancer.

I would like to thank everyone who contributed to this book. I thank Hugh Faulkner, M.D., a distinguished member of our international network of macrobiotic physicians, for contributing the Foreword, and for providing his personal case history. I also thank the contributors for writing their inspiring recovery stories and for granting permission to use them in the book. I thank my co-author, Edward Esko—who, more than fifteen years ago, edited our earliest publications on macrobiotics and cancer, and organized the first of many conferences on cancer and diet—for compiling the materials and adding insights based on years of experience as a macrobiotic teacher. I also thank Alex Jack, co-author of *The Cancer Prevention Diet*, for providing research and statistics used in the book, and Lawrence H. Kushi, Sc.D., a nutritional researcher at the University of Minnesota, for compiling information included in the chapter on macrobiotics and preventive nutrition. I appreciate the work of the editorial and production staffs, including Lynda Shoup of One Peaceful World, and Rudy Shur, Linda Comac, and the staff of Avery Publishing Group.

Michio Kushi
Brookline, Massachusetts

1

Cancer and Modern Civilization

A study of the macrobiotic diet's effect on cancer of the pancreas was reported on by medical researcher Gordon Saxe at the 1989 Macrobiotic Summer Conference held in Great Barrington, Massachusetts. Conducted in 1985 by the Tulane School of Public Health, the study attempted to find out whether persons with pancreatic cancer who adopted the macrobiotic diet survived longer than those who did not. The subjects of the study were a group of twenty-four pancreatic cancer patients who had practiced a macrobiotic diet for at least three months. The control group consisted of pancreatic cancer patients from the national tumor registry who were diagnosed during the same period. Among the twenty-four macrobiotic patients, the one-year survival rate was 54.2 percent (13/24), compared with 10.0 percent (950/9500) in the control group. Saxe told the conference that although not conclusive, these results were highly statistically significant.

Even though more research along these lines is urgently needed, the Tulane study suggests that a macrobiotically balanced diet may positively influence the outcome of existing cancers. Presently, many leading nutritional and public health agencies agree that a naturally balanced, low-fat diet along the lines of macrobiotics could help prevent or lower the risk of cancer, but this study is one of the first to suggest that diet has an influence on already established cancers.

This conclusion is supported by a growing body of anecdotal evidence. Over the years, my associates and I have worked with many exceptional cancer patients who overcame the odds and went on to lead normal, healthy, and productive lives. Hugh Faulkner, M.D., a former London physician who now lives in Italy, is an outstanding example. Dr. Faulkner was diagnosed with cancer of the pancreas in 1987. Being a physician, he was aware that medically there was little hope of recovery, and that the usual rate of survival after diagnosis of pancreatic cancer is two to four months. Dr. Faulkner and his wife, Marion, embarked on the macrobiotic way of life soon after the cancer was discovered, and by the autumn of 1988 medical tests showed "no evidence of cancer, no evidence of abnormality of any kind."

There are many exceptional cancer patients who, like Dr. Faulkner, have adopted macrobiotics and experienced a return to good health. In this book we introduce several of their remarkable and inspiring stories. Moreover, an increasing number of doctors and health care professionals in the United States and in other countries have adopted the macrobiotic way of life. My wife, Aveline, and I have presented seminars for doctors in Boston, Becket (Massachusetts), France, Yugoslavia, Hungary, and central Africa. Several hundred doctors are now part of an international network of macrobiotic physicians, many of whom recommend macrobiotics as a viable approach to health promotion and disease prevention. The macrobiotic physicians' network hopes to report scientific data by standardizing record-keeping among patients who practice macrobiotics. Hopefully, data such as this will stimulate further research and influence public health policy toward greater recognition of the role of diet in health.

THE MODERN HEALTH CRISIS

Over the past half century, medical science has conducted a massive campaign in an attempt to solve the problem of cancer. To date, this large-scale effort has not produced a solution. A May 1986 article entitled "Progress Against Cancer," published in the *New England Journal of Medicine*, summa-

Physician, Heal Thyself

Hugh Faulkner had never been happier. He had completed a successful career as a general practitioner in London and had retired to a beautiful old farmhouse in Italy. After returning to the countryside outside of Florence with his wife, Marion, the former London physician learned he had cancer of the pancreas.

"We both knew the diagnosis was more or less a death sentence," he recalled in an interview with *The Independent*, a British newspaper.

After her husband was referred to a surgeon who wanted to operate immediately, Marion asked, "What happens if he doesn't have surgery?" She was told, "He'll certainly obstruct." Bowel obstruction or difficulties with food absorption are common with pancreatic cancer, and Dr. Faulkner started to experience both. He underwent surgery to relieve the obstruction, but surgeons made no attempt to remove the cancer. In the hospital, after several days on liquids, he was put on solid foods again, "That day the lady from the kitchens came to see me," he recalls. "'Would you like steak and kidney pudding, dear?' she asked. I noticed we were given no advice at all on diet."

Meanwhile, a young woman who had given the Faulkners shiatsu treatments for back pain recommended macrobiotics. Dr. Faulkner recalled that during his career he had not been a conventional physician. "I used to refer my patients to people I thought could help them even if I thought they were 'alternative.' But I hadn't referred cases of incurable cancer. And I hadn't any real contact with alternative medicine. I'm not a believer; I'm congenitally skeptical."

After reading several books, Dr. Faulkner decided that macrobiotics might "help improve the quality of the months remaining to me." The usual rate of survival after diagnosis for pancreatic cancer is two to four months. It is rare to live even a year. "All our medical friends naturally assumed that I would die," Dr. Faulkner explains. "But by this time I'd decided that what I was afraid of was not death itself. It was the pain, the incontinence, the loss of autonomy when I became helpless that I dreaded."

Back in England, the Faulkners checked into a hospice—a center for the dying. While awaiting the end, they went to the Community Health Foundation, the macrobiotic center in London. A macrobiotic teacher who was visiting from Boston advised them on diet and encouraged them to see Michio Kushi for additional recommendations.

About six weeks later they met Michio during one of his European seminars. "Kushi was a small, slim, very modest man, with considerable charisma," Dr. Faulkner recalls. "It was all very warm and friendly and unmedical. Kushi spent a long time examining my skin texture—its appearance, elasticity, and color. Then I said, 'Well, can macrobiotics heal my cancer?'"

"'No,' said Kushi, 'but your body can. What we can do is advise you on a diet and way of life that will almost certainly make you feel much better, and give your body a chance to reject the cancer. We can't give you any guarantees—but we have plenty of evidence from cases like yours that it can work.'"

Although Dr. Faulkner was a little skeptical, Marion was enthusiastic, and they decided to try it. Returning to their farmhouse in Italy, the couple started cooking for themselves. The diet Michio recommended was a modified version of the standard macrobiotic diet. For breakfast, there was whole grain porridge and occasionally whole grain bread. Lunch included vegetable soup and tofu, tempeh, or another protein dish. Dinner consisted of pressure-cooked brown rice and vegetables and, occasionally, stewed fruit.

Dr. Faulkner's diarrhea went away, and he began to feel better. Marion also experienced improvement—she began to feel more energetic and confident. Visitors who came by to say farewell to the dying doctor were amazed to find him chopping wood and full of energy.

By the autumn of 1988, medical tests showed "no evidence of cancer, no evidence of abnormality of any kind." In London, some doctors questioned the initial diagnosis of cancer. Dr. Faulkner showed them his biopsy report and introduced them to his surgeon. They didn't want to believe and labeled his recovery "spontaneous regression."

Now, two and a half years later, Dr. Faulkner continues to thrive. He eats and sleeps well, entertains many visitors, and swims several times a week. He has also learned how to read music, play the jazz harmonica, and use a word processor. "I have a lot more energy than I've had in years."

"As an orthodox doctor, I myself wouldn't have thought of diet influencing the course of disease," Dr. Faulkner admits. "I'm now quite sure that we can learn a great deal from alternative medicine.

"The big change in macrobiotics was hope, however implausible. That, and the feeling that I was regaining control of my destiny."

Source: "A Doctor Heals Himself of Terminal Cancer," *One Peaceful World*, Autumn 1989.

rized current scientific thinking about present approaches to cancer: "We are losing the war against cancer, notwithstanding progress against several uncommon forms of the disease, improvements in palliation, and extension of the productive years of life. A shift in research emphasis, from research on treatment to research on prevention, seems necessary if substantial progress against cancer is to be forthcoming."

Among the possible avenues of prevention, dietary and lifestyle modifications are inexpensive and offer realistic hope of reducing the incidence of cancer. Yet, of the billions of dollars spent each year for cancer research, very little is channeled into the study of diet and cancer. This deficiency was cited more than ten years ago by the United States Congress in a report entitled *Nutrition Research Alternatives* prepared in 1978 by the Office of Technology Assessment. The conclusion is as valid today as it was then: "Federal human nutrition research programs have failed to deal with the changing health problems of the American people. Possibly the most productive and important area of nutrition research will be the identification of specific dietary links to chronic diseases, leading to methods of prevention."

At present, America and the rest of the modern world are in the midst of a crisis in health. The modern health crisis extends far beyond problems in the distribution of medical technology, the crisis in emergency care, or the astronomical cost of modern medicine itself. It is well known that the rates of cancer, heart disease, diabetes, osteoporosis, AIDS and immune deficiencies, Alzheimer's disease, and other degenerative disorders have been steadily increasing throughout the century, and in nearly all the world's populations. These increases have taken place even as medical science developed to its present level. At the turn of the century, for example, cancer affected one out of twenty-seven people in the United States. By 1950, the rate had jumped to one in eight; and by 1985, official estimates were that one out of three people would develop the disease.

If cancer keeps increasing at this rate, by the year 2000, every other person could ultimately develop it. By the year 2020, cancer could strike four out of five people, and, soon after that, virtually everyone. The figures are presented in Table 1.1.

Table 1.1.   **The Increasing Incidence of Cancer in the United States**

Year	Proportion of U.S. Population
1900	1 out of 27
1950	1 out of 8
1985	1 out of 3
Future Projections	
2000	1 out of 2
2020	4 out of 5
2030	virtually everyone

About 76 million Americans now living will eventually develop cancer, according to the American Cancer Society. Cancer will affect three out of four families in the United States. In 1990, approximately one million people were diagnosed with cancer. In addition, more than 600,000 cases of usually non-fatal skin cancer were diagnosed. The second leading cause of death in the United States, cancer claims more than 500,000 Americans each year. In the 1980s, there were over 4.5 million cancer deaths, nearly 9 million new cases, and 12 million people under medical care for cancer. About 1.5 million biopsies are performed each year.

As we can see, the modern health crisis, in which cancer is but one part, has the potential to affect everyone. The responsibility for finding and implementing solutions belongs to all of us, not just to those in the medical and scientific communities. A solution to cancer and the modern health crisis as a whole will emerge only through the cooperative effort of all people in society.

CANCER AND MODERN LIFE

The rise of cancer and other degenerative diseases during the twentieth century is a sign that something is wrong with modern life. The modern way of looking at the world may itself be problematic. Today, progress is viewed in materialistic terms, while intangible, spiritual values are often overlooked or short-changed. But this view is out of proportion with the nature of existence since the material world is tiny, almost insignificant, when compared with the invisible world of spirit.

A Doctor Looks at Macrobiotics

In December 1983, a close friend was found to have inoperable colon cancer that had spread to the liver. He was given just four to six months to live. Since there was then and, at this writing, still is, no known treatment for this disease once it has spread beyond the intestines, and since chemotherapy could, at best, offer only a possibility of temporary prolongation of life, he chose not to receive any medical treatment, but instead to try macrobiotics. He and his family followed the macrobiotic diet 100 percent, without any deviations, and became totally involved in the macrobiotic way of life. Almost every night his wife and son gave him a shiatsu massage. After three months of being on the macrobiotic diet, he began running, and by September of 1984, he ran half a marathon. In November 1985, a CAT scan showed no sign of cancer, and my friend's present health is excellent. This is truly astounding in view of the fact that there is only one recorded case of spontaneous regression of metastatic colon cancer.

In light of this spectacular regression from cancer, I began research into macrobiotics in June 1984. This included: (1) following a number of patients with cancer who had chosen macrobiotics (with or without chemotherapy); (2) questioning as many patients (or their relatives) as possible who had sought macrobiotic counseling, for either pancreatic cancer or brain tumor; (3) sending detailed questionnaires to people who felt they had had a serious illness and had done much better with macrobiotics; and (4) documenting in the appropriate scientific fashion a number of cases of medically incurable, terminal patients with biopsy-proven cancer who had followed macrobiotics and who had completely recovered from advanced cancer.

The number of patients in this last group is small, and although this does not prove that macrobiotics can bring about recovery from cancer, it indicates that for the patient who cannot be offered hope medically, macrobiotics is certainly worth a try.

Source: Vivien Newbold, M.D., *Macrobiotics: An Approach to the Achievement of Health, Happiness, and Harmony, Doctors Look at Macrobiotics*, Japan Publications, 1988.

Not only is the physical world tiny in comparison with the world of spirit, but as modern physics has discovered, matter is actually composed of energy and is constantly changing. Our perceptions trick us into believing that the world has a fixed or unchanging nature, but reality is not like that. Our bodies, for example, are composed of energy and are not static and inert, but dynamic and changing. Today's "self" is very different from yesterday's "self" and tomorrow's "self." The changing nature of human life is obvious to parents who have watched their children grow. Moreover, we don't stop changing after we reach physical maturity: our body, mind, and consciousness constantly change and develop throughout life.

There is nothing static, fixed, or permanent in this universe. If we are able to recognize this, then we are more likely to be open to the possibility of making constructive changes in our lives, and to the possibility of discovering new dimensions of health and healing. Reorienting our priorities to reflect the true nature of existence can help us relieve stress and mobilize our innate capacities for self-healing.

I often meet people who, although they know they need to change their diets and eat well, say that the demands of their careers prevent them from doing so. They sometimes say, "I know I should eat well, but I don't have time to cook," or "I travel a lot and need to eat in restaurants." I tell them that there is nothing wrong with having a successful career, but that success should not come at the expense of their health and well-being. Health is the foundation of life; and if we lose it, we lose the ability to be successful and to function normally.

Parallel to the triumph of materialism is the trend toward increasing alienation from nature. Modern people are rapidly moving toward a totally artificial way of life. However, regardless of what direction society takes, life cannot exist without the solar system or the Earth, or without air, water, or vegetation. By cutting ourselves off from nature and polluting or destroying the environment, we are undercutting the very foundation of life and health.

The quality of food offers a good example. Our ancestors appreciated the simple, natural taste and texture of brown bread, brown rice, and other whole, natural foods. Now, in order to appease the senses or satisfy the demand for convenience, brown rice is refined and polished into white rice, whole-wheat bread has been replaced by white bread, and fresh garden vegetables are frozen or canned. These foods lack the natural balance of energy and nutrients found in their unprocessed counterparts, and are inadequate for maintaining human health.

At the same time, a huge industry has developed that enhances sensory appeal by adding artificial colorings, flavorings, and texturing agents to our daily foods. Food is not the only thing that has become more artificial. Over the last fifty years, this trend has been extended to clothing, building materials, furniture, kitchen utensils, and other items essential for daily living. As many people have discovered, however, artificial conveniences such as microwave ovens, computer display terminals, electric appliances, and fluorescent lights can have deleterious effects on human health.

Cancer is only one result of an unnatural lifestyle and way of eating. However, instead of considering the larger environmental, societal, and dietary causes of cancer, most research—with the exception of epidemiological or large-scale population studies—is oriented in the opposite direction: viewing the disease microscopically as a disorder of individual cells.

Cancer originates long before the formation of a tumor, and is rooted in our lifestyle, including the foods we consume. When cancer is finally discovered, however, modern treatments focus almost exclusively on the tumor, while the patient's diet and lifestyle are often ignored. Often, the foods most associated with the patient's cancer are served to the patient in the hospital. In many cases, patients are told that diet has nothing to do with cancer so "eat whatever you want." But since the cause is not changed, the cancer frequently recurs, and is met by another round of treatment in what is often an unsuccessful attempt to control only the symptoms of the disease. As we can see, this approach deals with effects, not causes.

In order to control cancer, we need to see beyond its obvious symptoms. We need to identify and, hopefully, change the underlying factors that cause these symptoms to appear, beginning with the patient's dietary and lifestyle habits. We also need to see beyond the individual patient. The orientation of the food industry, the quality of modern agriculture, and the

Skin Cancer Linked to Fluorescent Lights

In a study published in *The Lancet*, researchers at the London School of Hygiene and Tropical Medicine discovered that fluorescent lighting in the office was associated with a two to two-and-a-half-fold increase in the risk of melanoma, a particularly virulent form of skin cancer that is increasing in incidence in the United States and other countries. The researchers reached this conclusion after questioning 274 female melanoma patients and 549 matched controls in Australia about certain lifestyle factors that might increase their risk of cancer. A review of other data collected on 27 male melanoma patients and 35 controls found an even stronger correlation—a 4.4-fold increase for exposure of 10 years or more.

Source: J. A. Treichel, *Science News*, Volume 122, August 28, 1982.

increasingly sedentary nature of modern life all have a direct bearing on the problem of cancer.

From the macrobiotic view, then, cancer is a symptom of modern society itself: its artificial farming practices, its unhealthful diet, and its preoccupation with short-term gain at the expense of long-term health and well-being. In the chapters that follow, we explore ways in which to change our diet, lifestyle, and way of thinking in order to turn away from cancer and toward genuine health.

2

A Holistic Approach
to Lifestyle

Cancer does not result from factors that are beyond our control. It is a product of the choices we make daily—including the foods we choose to eat—and does not strike at random. The primary factors that lead to cancer are under our control. Cancer is a preventable disease, if we change our habits early enough. But, beyond prevention, evidence is mounting that lifestyle changes guided by macrobiotic principles can improve the prognosis for cancer and aid in the recovery of health.

In order to establish health, we need to change the principal factors that cause cancer to develop. It is important to address the issue of health from a holistic perspective; that is, to consider health to be the natural outcome of harmony in the whole person—mind, body, and spirit. The macrobiotic approach aims at restoring these aspects to a state of harmony with each other and with nature, primarily through adjustments in diet, lifestyle, and way of thinking.

Sickness is actually a sign that some aspect of our daily lives is causing us to become out of alignment with nature. In one sense, it offers an opportunity to step back and reassess our thinking and actions, and to, hopefully, make the necessary corrections. In macrobiotics, this type of evaluation is known as self-reflection, and it is an essential part of the recovery process.

Most of the time, our day-to-day thinking consists of thoughts and images that arise in response to the stimulation we receive from our immediate environment. Our ongoing internal dialogue includes thoughts such as: "I hope I get the promotion I was asking for," or "I'm looking forward to my vacation in Jamaica," or "I wonder who will win the big game tonight?" However, each of us has a deeper level of awareness that transcends the superficial levels of consciousness. Here are the understanding, the dreams, and the images that we all have as human beings, and not just as people who work in an office or who manage a household budget. This deeper awareness often surfaces during times of crisis, and provides the basis for self-reflection and change. It functions as an internal compass or inner guide that helps keep us aligned with nature. If, for example, someone is told of a life-threatening illness, or is facing a life-or-death, "to-be-or-not-to-be" situation, then this deeper mind starts to emerge. From deep inside, a person in this situation will start to think, "I don't care about my office work or other superficial things. What shall I do as a human being?"

This deeper consciousness, or intuition, alerts us to potentially destructive habits or patterns of behavior, and includes the instinct for survival, or self-preservation. It also motivates us to change these habits. Beyond differences in nationality, race, religion, or social standing, we all have this basic common sense.

Mobilizing this deeper level of awareness is the key to recovering from illness. Intuition does not mean day-to-day consciousness or learned knowledge, which often obscures deeper awareness and obstructs positive action. Intuition is the unlearned, spontaneous awareness of the order of nature and the way to live in harmony with that order. It is the foundation for a long and healthy life on this planet.

Meditation offers a simple and practical method to dissolve stress, quiet the mind, and mobilize your intuition. To practice simple meditation, do the following:

1. Find a quiet place and sit in a relaxed and comfortable position.

2. Raise your arms upward toward the ceiling and hold them there for several moments. Then tilt your head back so that you are looking up. Keep your head in this position for several seconds, and then lower your arms to their normal position. Return your head to its normal position a moment later. This simple stretching exercise helps straighten your spine and allows energy from the environment to flow more smoothly through your body. Do each step in a continuous sequence and repeat the entire procedure several times.
3. With your spine straight and your shoulders and elbows relaxed, let your hands rest comfortably in your lap.
4. Close your eyes and begin to breathe naturally and quietly. Breathe in a normal, relaxed fashion.
5. While you are breathing in this manner, let your mind become quiet, relaxed, and free of distracting thoughts. Sit this way for several minutes, breathing naturally and keeping your mind still and quiet.
6. To complete your meditation, slowly open your eyes and let your consciousness return to a normal waking state.

You can also practice visualization, or creative imaging, while meditating. Visualizing more positive images of health is preferable to visualizing images that focus on sickness or internal struggle. To practice visualization, begin to meditate as above. When you have reached step four, form an image of yourself as a healthy and happy person. Don't dwell on your illness; see yourself as you would like to be. Concentrate on this image for several minutes and then let your mind return to a peaceful, quiet state. Then complete your meditation as above. Positive visualization reduces stress and inspires hope for the future. Your daily life can then become the process through which you actualize this positive, healthy image of yourself.

THE ROLE OF LOVE IN HEALING

One of the surprising things that our intuition reveals is that love, or the attraction and harmony of opposites, is the ordering principle of nature. I call this "surprising" because much of our human experience seems to contradict this basic truth.

Love is based on the attraction of opposites such as male and female, adults and children, the self and others. The invisible force that brings men and women together also causes the planets to revolve around the sun, hydrogen and oxygen atoms to be attracted to each other to form molecules of water, the seasons to change, and flowers to blossom.

Love is one of the most potent forces in healing. It liberates a tremendous amount of energy, and brings our total being into harmony with the universe. Love enables the body's powers of natural healing to operate with fewer impediments.

The fear and anxiety that often accompany illness have the opposite effect. Although they sometimes act as a driving force for positive change, in the long-run, negative emotions deplete energy and impede our capacity for natural healing.

These responses to sickness arise because we lack an understanding of the cause of our problems. If, for example, we view sickness as being caused by an external factor—such as a virus or bacterium—rather than by our own lifestyle and actions, we lose sight of our personal responsibility in causing our sickness. Our illness then becomes an "enemy" that must be fought and vanquished, rather than a signal from nature that some aspect of our lifestyle is in need of change. In thinking this way, we may forfeit the opportunity to actively participate in creating our health. We assume a passive role and think that health can be restored by having things "done" to us by others, rather than by making constructive efforts on our own.

Unfortunately, modern thinking about disease is often based on fear and hostility, even as it becomes increasingly clear that cancer, heart disease, and other chronic illnesses are caused by personal lifestyle choices and not by outside agents such as bacteria or viruses. Not only is sickness an enemy, but in the modern view, the body itself is a battleground. The immune system, for example, is thought of as "defending" the body "against" disease; while immune cells are often described as "soldiers" that "battle" cancer cells or "invading" microorganisms.

In the macrobiotic view, the body's immune response is based on the process of natural attraction and harmony that is found throughout the universe. The antibodies secreted by

Finding the Macrobiotic Way

In November 1980, Bonnie Kramer, a twenty-seven-year-old mother from Torrington, Connecticut, felt discomfort under her arm. She discovered a pea-sized ball that "seemed to float" when touched, but she was not overly concerned about it. She underwent a mammography the following February and the results were negative.

During the winter, the lump went through periods of increasing and decreasing size, and she started to experience constant pain in her left breast along with fatigue and a milky white discharge from the nipple. Her breasts were enlarged and tender. She also had an unusual number of colds and flu.

A biopsy in February 1982, revealed cancer, and soon afterward Bonnie entered Winsted Memorial Hospital in Connecticut for the removal of her left breast and several lymph nodes under her arm. She also began chemotherapy and was scheduled to undergo six weeks of radiation. The side effects were not severe, although she was irritable at times, lost some hair, and became nauseated after each treatment. Bonnie completed her treatments in March 1983, and was considered by her doctors to be free of cancer. However, periodic bone and liver scans were advised as a precaution. Feeling better, she took a job as a director of social services at a skilled nursing facility and helped raise funds for the American Cancer Society.

Three years later, in April 1986, while playing Wiffle ball with her son, Bonnie felt a pull in her lower back. The pain continued off and on, and by early 1987 had become unbearable. "The pain returned with a vengeance," she recalls. "It just would not go away, and the nurses at work became very concerned. The pain radiated to my face. With each menstrual cycle, I was bloated, suffering with intense cramps." She underwent a bone scan that revealed tumors on her pelvis and upper back. Her doctors advised radiation and aggressive chemotherapy. Bonnie was "numbed to speechlessness" at the news, and "couldn't stop crying." As she recalls, "I had to deal with this; that's all I knew. I prayed for strength and guidance in the midst of all this drama. Then suddenly, out of nowhere, it hit me! Honestly, just like that the answer came. I knew from my readings that more and more was being learned about nutrition and cancer. I remembered my sister's telling me about an article she had read several years before, concerning a doctor whose cancer went into remission through a change in diet. It didn't seem relevant to me then, but, suddenly, now it did. 'O my God!' I thought,

'That's what I need to do—find out more about this diet, but how?'"

Bonnie's friend went to a local health food store and bought a copy of Michio Kushi's *The Macrobiotic Way* for her to read. She found it completely logical but overwhelming. She went to the health food store and bought staple foods and stopped eating meat, sugar, and dairy food. She also underwent radiation therapy and a hysterectomy. After recovering from surgery, Bonnie decided to attend the Macrobiotic Way of Life Seminar presented by the Kushi Institute (K.I.).

Bonnie supplemented her practice of macrobiotics by taking weekly cooking classes with Sara Lapenta, a K.I. cooking teacher who lived nearby. By May 1987, a blood test revealed that Bonnie's enzyme levels had returned to normal. A bone scan in September showed that the tumors had greatly decreased in size. A friend who worked in the radiation unit at the hospital told her that she had never seen a report like that before. In September 1988, another bone scan revealed the presence of scar tissue but no tumors. Her doctor told her that her remission might have been due to the surgery and radiation, but that macrobiotics may have also helped her. By August 1988, a bone scan produced a totally normal result, with no tumors or scar tissue. Her doctor was now very impressed and fully supportive of her macrobiotic lifestyle.

Bonnie describes her macrobiotic experience: "I noticed immediate changes in myself and my son Ben, who joined in my meals for the first summer. Our allergies seemed to disappear and Ben no longer got strep throat. We felt stronger, more energetic, more organized, and very well. I had good spirits and stable moods. As my confidence increased, so did the sense of inner peace. I loved feeling at one with nature, at one with God."

Bonnie is now preparing to open a macrobiotic center in her area. Believing that "happiness is real only if it can be shared with others," she would like to help people in her area through classes, food, and guidance. She has dedicated herself to realizing one peaceful world and is grateful to have found a way to "help make this concept a reality."

Source: "A Mother Heals Breast Cancer: Change in Diet Aids Remission of Tumors and Metastases to the Bone," *One Peaceful World,* Spring, 1990.

immune cells actually complement and make a balance with cancer cells, viruses, or other potentially harmful substances. Antibodies have an opposite polarity to these cells and neutralize their extreme or excessive qualities, thus keeping the body in a state of healthy equilibrium. In other words, the immune response is a process of natural harmony, not war. When we are healthy, the immune system functions efficiently and we remain free of sickness. When our overall condition deteriorates, the immune system loses the ability to neutralize these substances and we become sick.

Cancer, heart disease, and other modern degenerative illnesses are diseases of overconsumption. To a large extent, they are a product of the excessive struggle for prosperity and convenience. Modern life is highly competitive and creates a great deal of stress. It also revolves around patterns of excessive consumption. The regular consumption of animal protein and fat, for example, is at the heart of the modern notion of prosperity. In the past, meat and other animal foods were often too expensive for the average person to eat regularly. They were foods of the rich, and today are still associated with wealth and status. This dietary pattern, however, underlies the modern epidemic of cancer, heart disease, and other degenerative illnesses.

As long as we cling to the notion that sickness is an enemy, or that human life is ruled by a struggle for survival, a solution to the problem of cancer will remain elusive. This view obscures our awareness of the peaceful, natural process of harmony that occurs in the human body and throughout nature. There is no war taking place in our bodies or in the universe. Sickness is not our enemy. The modern notion of "cell wars" is simply a projection of our modern imagination and not a reflection of the way things are.

The order of the universe is the order of balance and harmony, or in other words, love. In order to be healthy, we need to bring our view of life into alignment with the natural order. We must learn to love other people and ourselves, and to regard sickness not as an enemy, but as an opportunity to discover a deeper meaning of health. Love, appreciation, and acceptance are basic to health and to being at peace with ourselves and the world around us.

RECONNECTING WITH NATURE

When we stop to think about it, many aspects of modern living have caused us to lose touch with nature. That is due, in part, to the notion that human beings can somehow conquer, alter, or improve nature without having to worry about the consequences. This paradigm is based on the incorrect assumption that human beings are more powerful than nature, and is evidence of a fundamental lack of respect for the natural environment and for the integrity of the human body. The results of thinking this way can be disastrous.

To recover health, we need to cultivate the opposite attitude. We need to appreciate nature as the source of our lives and reaffirm our connection with that source. Personal health cannot be separated from planetary health. This involves becoming aware of the environmental consequences of our actions and sensitive to what our bodies are trying to tell us. Actually, we receive messages from our bodies all the time that alert us to imbalance and signal us to make corrective changes. Common illnesses such as headaches, colds and flu, digestive upsets, fatigue, skin rashes, and others are actually signals that our eating, drinking, and lifestyle as a whole are out of order. However, instead of heeding these messages and making the necessary changes, most people take medications designed to make the problem "go away," while continuing on as before. This allows them to avoid dealing with the problem at the moment. But, by not changing, they are increasing the likelihood that the problem will reappear or that a more serious health problem will develop in the future.

The relation between man and nature is like that between the embryo and the placenta. The placenta nourishes, supports, and sustains the developing embryo. It would be quite bizarre if the embryo were to seek to destroy this protector organism. Likewise, it is a matter of common sense that we should strive to preserve the environment upon which we depend for life itself. Over the last century, however, we have pursued the opposite course and have steadily aggravated the contamination of our soil, water, and air.

The degradation of the environment has direct consequences for our personal health. There are 4.5 million known toxic chemicals with thousands of new chemicals being syn-

(the word "molar" is from the Latin word meaning "mill-stone") are ideally suited for crushing the tough plant fibers that are found in whole cereal grains, beans, seeds, and other complex carbohydrate foods.

There are also eight front incisors and four canine teeth. The word "incisor" comes from the Latin word meaning "to cut into," and these teeth are well suited for cutting vegetables. The four canine teeth can be used for tearing animal foods, but are not sharply pointed in everyone. People who live in societies that consume little or no animal food often do not develop pointed canines.

Using the teeth as a model, we can conclude that, ideally, about five parts of the human diet would consist of whole grains, beans, seeds, and other tough plant fibers; two parts, local vegetables; and up to one part, animal food. The optimum ratio of plant to animal food is about seven to one.

Human intestines are another clue to ideal eating patterns. Our intestines are long and convoluted compared with those of carnivorous (meat-eating) animals. The digestive system of carnivorous animals promotes rapid food transit; as a result, the toxic byproducts of decaying animal flesh are less likely to accumulate. But in our case, a diet high in animal foods transits slowly through the digestive system, allowing toxins to accumulate throughout the body. Ultimately, this results in a variety of disorders, including cancer. It is to our advantage to eat primarily plant foods. The correlation between consumption of animal fat and protein and cancer of the colon is evidence that a diet based on animal foods is not well-suited to human needs.

ADVANTAGES OF TRADITIONAL DIETS

The modern highly refined, high-fat, low-fiber diet became widespread largely over the last 100 years, and includes many items that were unknown in the past. Humanity's traditional staples—whole cereal grains, beans, and fresh local vegetables—are no longer consumed as principal foods. The rising incidence of cancer and other degenerative diseases in the twentieth century parallels these changes in the human diet.

Over the last three generations, cancer has risen by 800

The Changing American Diet

According to surveys conducted by the U.S. Department of Agriculture, the American diet has changed radically in this century. Consumption of traditional staples, such as grains and their products, beans, and fresh vegetables and fruit, plummeted; the intake of meat, poultry, sugar, cheese, soft drinks, and processed foods skyrocketed. USDA surveys show that from 1910 to 1976 per capita intake of grains fell 51 percent. Consumption of corn, the traditional staple of North and South America, fell 85 percent and consumption of other traditional staples such as rye fell 78 percent; wheat, 48 percent; barley, 66 percent; buckwheat, 98 percent. The intake of beans fell 46 percent, fresh vegetables, 23 percent; fresh fruit, 33 percent. During the same period the intake of beef rose 72 percent; cheese, 322 percent; poultry, 194 percent; canned vegetables, 320 percent; frozen vegetables, 1,650 percent; processed fruit, 556 percent; yogurt, 300 percent; ice cream, 852 percent; corn syrup, 761 percent; sugar, 29 percent; saccharine, 300 percent; soft drinks, 2,638 percent. The per capita intake of artificial food colors added to the diet has risen 995 percent since 1940, the first year that consumption of chemical additives and preservatives was recorded.

percent, according to data compiled by the National Center for Health Statistics. Today nearly one out of three Americans dies of cancer. At the turn of the century, one out of twenty-seven died of cancer. A National Cancer Institute study on cancer research reported that in the 1830s, when cancer statistics were first recorded in Paris, researchers noted that about one in fifty died from cancer. Thus cancer has increased fifteen-fold in the West over the last two centuries. This period corresponds with major changes in our way of eating, including the widespread refining of flour and overall decrease of grains in the diet; increased consumption of meat, sugar, and dairy products; daily consumption of tropical foods and beverages in temperate zones (and vice-versa); the introduction of chemical agriculture; the invention of synthetic foods and chemical additives; high-technology food

AREAS WITH THE EARTH'S LOWEST CANCER:

processing such as canning and freezing; and the introduction of electric cooking and refrigeration, and microwave ovens.

Whole grains have traditionally been known in all cultures as the staff of life. The decline and fall of organically grown whole grains since the beginning of the modern age in the seventeenth century parallels the rise and spread of cancer. Investigating this relationship is a major area for future study among medical historians and cancer specialists.

Despite the spread of refined and synthetic foods around the world, cooked whole grains, beans, and vegetables are still eaten as main foods in many cultures today. For example, corn tortillas and black beans are the staple foods in Central America; rice and soybean products are eaten throughout Southeast Asia; whole and cracked wheat and chickpeas are daily fare in the Middle East. These regions have the lowest rates of cancer in the world. Recent international surveys comparing the rate of cancer mortality in males in forty-four countries found the least cancer in countries where traditional dietary patterns still prevail, such as El Salvador, Thailand, and Egypt. In comparison, European nations registered the highest incidence, and the United States, Canada, and Australia were also found to be in the upper range. In these parts of the world, the modern diet has all but replaced traditional ways of eating.

As we point out in *The Cancer Prevention Diet*, there are still a few traditional societies around the world in which cancer is rare or unknown. These include some Native American tribes, certain non-Israeli Jewish communities in the Middle East, various African cultures, and the Hunza in Pakistan. Substantial medical literature already exists on the relative absence of cancer in primitive society. In *The Natural History of Cancer* (William Wood & Co., 1908), Dr. W. Roger Williams, a Fellow of the Royal College of Surgery in London, surveyed field reports from British medical doctors in Asia and Africa and found that cancer was non-existent in cultures where people were eating primarily grains, seeds, tubers, and other vegetable foods. Almost eighty-five years ago, Dr. Williams concluded that in the West, cancer was a disease of "overnutrition," caused mainly by excessive intake of protein from animal sources.

In *Studies in Deficiency Disease* (1921), Sir Robert Mc-

Carrison, another British surgeon, reported that cancer was unknown among the Hunza who ate a daily diet consisting of whole-wheat chapatis, barley, and buckwheat supplemented by leafy green vegetables, beans and legumes, apricots, and very small amounts of animal food. In 1927, as director of Nutritional Research in India, McCarrison began a series of laboratory experiments to test whether the Hunza diet was chiefly responsible for the absence of degenerative disease in this isolated region of India. He fed one group of rats the Hunza diet and a control group the regular Indian diet high in refined white rice, sugar, and spices. The tests showed that rats fed the Hunza diet high in whole grains remained healthy and free of all disease, while those on the processed diet contracted cysts, abscesses, heart disease, and cancer.

In *Refined Carbohydrate Foods and Disease* (Academic Press, 1975) and *Eat Right—To Keep Healthy and Enjoy Life* (Arco, 1979), British surgeon Denis Burkitt (a world-famous cancer specialist after whom Burkitt's Lymphoma is named) concluded that most cancers came to Africa with imported modern food and that Africans who ate a traditional high-fiber diet remained cancer-free. Dr. Albert Schweitzer also associated the appearance of cancer in West Africa with the adoption of refined foodstuffs. In his medical writings he singles out chemical salt, which replaced natural sea salt in the local diet, as a chief contributing factor.

Before the remaining few cancer-free societies disappear altogether, scientists should examine traditional patterns of agriculture, food preparation and cooking methods, and patterns of eating to discover the nutritional factors that may contribute to the absence of cancer and other degenerative disease.

HARMONY WITH THE ENVIRONMENT

A natural, ecologically balanced diet fulfills several criteria. For one, it is environmentally friendly, which means that it does not contribute to the degradation of the environment or waste valuable natural resources. The principal foods in an environmentally friendly diet are produced by sustainable, chemical-free agriculture, and return more energy than it

FOODS TO EAT BASED ON WEATER ZONES:
NORTH(COLD) TEMPERATE(MILD)TROPICAL(HOT)

takes to produce them. On an individual level, an ecologically balanced diet promotes health by harmonizing our condition with our immediate environment.

For thousands of years people ate the foods produced in their local environment. People in temperate zones ate the foods of temperate zones: whole grains, beans, fresh seasonal vegetables and fruits, and other products of their regional agriculture. Eating foods from the same climate makes it easier to create a balance with our immediate environment. Traditionally, for example, the Eskimo and other people in the Far North based their diets around fish and other animal foods found in the Arctic region. Vegetable foods were scarce, and a diet high in animal protein and fat helped them to strike a balance with their extreme climate. Following this principle, people in tropical regions lived on the unique plant and animal species found there. In India, for example, people naturally adopted a vegetarian or semivegetarian way of eating because minimizing the intake of animal food makes it easier to adapt to a hot climate.

Not only did foods vary from one climate to another, but so did traditional methods of cooking and food processing. For people in colder regions, food is an important source of heat. People in northern latitudes naturally cook their dishes thoroughly and include a higher percentage of animal protein, salt, and fat in their diets. In warmer regions, where lighter cooking is appropriate, people eat a larger volume of fresh foods and lightly cooked dishes and include less animal food and salt in their diets.

The shift to the modern diet blurred distinctions that for centuries had been rooted in the unique climate and environment of each region. Today, most Americans, Europeans, Japanese, and Soviets eat large amounts of meat and dairy products that are suited to a colder, semipolar climate. In addition, they eat fruits and vegetables native to the tropics, refined sugar and spices from the tropics, and cola beverages, coffee, and other stimulants prepared from tropical ingredients. This way of eating in a temperate zone goes against the *SUGAR* ecological order and, sooner or later, leads to ill health.

With a high intake of extremes like meat and sugar, people tend to overlook their traditional staples. Grains and beans today are fed to livestock and then eaten in the form of animal

90% OF U.S. GRAIN
IS FED TO ANIMALS.

food rather than being eaten directly. Forty percent of the world's grain (including ninety percent of American grain) is fed to cattle or other livestock to produce meat, poultry, dairy food, or other animal food. This highly inefficient practice not only depletes our human resources—in the form of increasing degenerative illness—but also depletes the earth's natural resources.

HARMONY WITH THE CHANGING SEASONS

Varying our selection of foods and cooking methods to reflect seasonal changes is an important aspect of eating a naturally balanced diet. During the winter, for example, we naturally seek hearty, warming foods, while in summer, quick, lightly cooked dishes are appealing. Also, cold weather tends to increase our appetite, while hot weather diminishes it. To a certain extent, people intuitively change their diet from season to season, but if we understand how to adjust our cooking and selection of foods, the transition can be much easier. This is especially important today since modern diets are often monotonously standardized throughout the year. Modern dietary habits cause us to lose touch with the cycles of nature and set in motion an accelerating spiral of ill health. Today, people eat barbecued ribs in the heat of the summer and frozen yogurt and ice cream in the middle of winter. These habits reflect an insensitivity to the subtleties of seasonal change, and have contributed to the rise of chronic illness.

The intake of ice cream, soft drinks, orange juice, and other chilled beverages in autumn and winter is one reason why people in temperate regions develop colds and flu during those seasons. These items cause fewer symptoms during the hot, dry weather of summer, but as the weather turns colder, they create a greater degree of imbalance between the body and the surrounding environment. As a result, the body seeks to discharge them.

Discharge can take many forms, including sneezing, coughing, chills and fever, and various intestinal symptoms. When handled properly—by not interfering with the natural process of discharge, for example—symptoms like these can be beneficial. They prevent excess from building up inside the body

ACUTE LEUKEMIA

Living and Loving

The summer of 1982 was a typical one for Doug Blampied, an insurance executive from Concord, New Hampshire. There was only a slight hint of his being a bit more tired and run-down than usual. Doug's end-of-summer plans were capped off with a sailing trip around Nantucket and Martha's Vineyard with his wife, Nancy. The trip was enjoyable, and Doug felt rested and refreshed. When he returned home, however, he couldn't quite get his energy level back to normal. Coming down with what he thought was a flu or virus, he went on with work as usual. When his fever wouldn't go down, he finally decided to see a doctor. After a routine checkup, he got dressed and returned home to bed.

Six hours later the phone rang. It was the doctor's office, and the message was urgent—get to the hospital immediately. With questions and fears racing through their minds, Doug and Nancy quickly packed and headed for the hospital, where a battery of tests was performed, including a painful bone marrow extraction.

The tests showed that Doug had acute myelogenous leukemia. Cancer of the spinal fluid was also discovered. Soon afterward, he started chemotherapy at a hospital in nearby Hanover. A Hickman catheter was implanted into his chest. It consisted of a plastic tube that was inserted into a vein leading to the heart. The catheter allowed the chemotherapy to be administered and blood to be withdrawn without repeated injections.

The chemotherapy caused a variety of side effects. Doug would wake up in the morning nauseated. When he tried to eat, he would usually vomit, sometimes as often as five times a day. He forced himself out of bed to bathe and use the toilet, only to fall back to bed, sick and exhausted. He lost his hair, became very thin, and was listless and weak. He was unable to do much for himself except eat, sleep, and get out of bed once a day with assistance.

Although doctors cautioned the family that Doug's chances for recovery were slight, Doug never lost the will to live. Several times his condition became so tenuous that the doctors told Nancy to make preparations for his death. Doug recalls, "Even though I felt unbelievably horrible, I didn't succumb to the idea of quitting. I had too much to do and wasn't finished with living yet. I would look at my wife and children and know I hadn't done all the things with them I wanted to do. I made up my mind to overcome this, whatever it took."

After a month and a half in the hospital, Doug began to show

MENTAL ATTITUDE

some improvement and was sent home. Over the next eight months, he received chemotherapy at home and continued to experience side effects, including high fevers. He was strong enough to return to work early in 1983, and monthly checkups showed his cancer was in remission, which meant that less than 25 percent of his cells were leukemic. If the percentage were to go higher, he would need to return to the hospital for additional chemotherapy.

In April of 1983, Doug underwent a bone marrow harvest. A team of doctors from Johns Hopkins University went to New Hampshire to perform the procedure, which was then being done at only a few hospitals in the United States. The first step in this painful process was the extraction of bone marrow from the spine. A hole was drilled into the bone and the marrow was extracted with a special instrument. The marrow was then treated with antibodies, frozen, and stored.

In the early 1980s, it was rare for a patient with Doug's type of cancer to survive a second remission for longer than six months. This meant that if the cancer came back, and went into remission again due to treatment, the prospects for long-term survival were slim. In Doug's case, if the remission were lost, the doctors planned to do a series of chemical and radiation treatments to kill the cells around the cancer. Then the previously harvested bone marrow, treated with antibodies, would be placed into his body.

A checkup just two months after the bone marrow harvest revealed that Doug's cancer count was again rising. Both Doug and Nancy were devastated. His doctor suggested going ahead with the bone marrow transplant, and advised against further chemotherapy since Doug was already in a weakened condition. He told Doug that even with chemotherapy, he would probably live only six months.

The bone marrow transplant also offered little hope. Doug and Nancy researched the success rate and found that out of the fifty or so patients who had been treated with the procedure at a leading medical center, only a handful were still alive. With little hope from either treatment, Doug and Nancy agonized over their decision. After much deliberation, they decided to forgo the transplant.

At a support group meeting, Doug was introduced to a copy of *Recalled by Life* by Anthony Sattilaro, M.D., and Tom Monte. It told the story of a doctor whose terminal metastatic prostate cancer went into remission after he adopted a macrobiotic diet. Encouraged by the possibility that macrobiotics might improve his condition, Doug journeyed to Brookline, Massachusetts,

Fruit or fruit desserts, including fresh, dried, and cooked fruits, may also be served two or three times per week. Local and organically grown fruits are preferred. If you live in a temperate climate, avoid tropical and semitropical fruit and eat, instead, temperate-climate fruits such as apples, pears, plums, peaches, apricots, berries, and melons. Frequent use of fruit juice is not advisable. However, depending on your condition, occasional consumption in warmer weather may be appropriate.

Lightly roasted seeds and nuts—pumpkin, sesame, and sunflower seeds, peanuts, walnuts, and pecans—may be enjoyed from time to time as a snack.

Rice syrup, barley malt, amazake, and mirin may be used as sweeteners; brown rice vinegar or umeboshi vinegar may be used occasionally for a sour taste.

Beverages

Recommended daily beverages include roasted bancha twig tea, roasted brown rice tea, roasted barley tea, dandelion tea, and cereal grain coffee. Any traditional tea that does not have an aromatic fragrance or a stimulating effect can be used. You may also drink a moderate amount of water (preferably spring or well water of good quality) but not iced.

Foods to Minimize or Avoid for Optimal Health

In a temperate climate, the following foods and beverages are best avoided for optimal health:

☐ Meat, animal fat, eggs, poultry, dairy products (including butter, yogurt, ice cream, milk, and cheese), refined sugars, chocolate, molasses, honey, other simple sugars and foods treated with them, and vanilla.

☐ Tropical or semitropical fruits and fruit juices, soda, artificially flavored drinks and beverages, coffee, colored tea,

and all aromatic or stimulating teas such as mint or pep-
permint tea.

☐ All artificially colored, preserved, sprayed, or chemically
treated foods. All refined and polished grains, flours,
and their derivatives. Mass-produced foods including all
canned, frozen, and irradiated foods. Hot spices, any aromatic, stimulating food or food accessory, artificial vinegar, and strong alcoholic beverages.

Additional Suggestions

Cooking oil should be vegetable quality only. To improve your
health, it is preferable to use only unrefined sesame or corn
oil in moderate amounts.

☐ Salt should be naturally processed sea salt. Traditional,
non-chemical shoyu or tamari soy sauce and miso may
also be used as seasonings. Use all seasonings in
moderation.

☐ Recommended condiments include:
  • Gomashio (12 to 18 parts roasted sesame seeds to 1
    part roasted sea salt)
  • Pickles (made using bran, miso, tamari soy sauce, sea
    salt), sauerkraut
  • Sea vegetable powder (kelp, kombu, wakame, and
    other sea vegetables)
  • Sesame sea vegetable powder
  • Tekka (selected root vegetables are sauteed with dark
    sesame oil and seasoned with soybean or hatcho
    miso)
  • Tamari soy sauce or shoyu (moderate use, for a mild
    flavor, only in cooking)
  • Umeboshi plums (pickled plums)

☐ You may eat regularly, two or three times per day, as
much as you want, provided the proportions are correct
and chewing is thorough. Avoid eating for approximately
three hours before sleeping.

☐ Proper cooking is very important for health. Everyone
should learn to cook either by attending classes or under
the guidance of an experienced macrobiotic cook. The

recipes included in the chapters that follow, along with those in the cookbooks listed in the bibliography, may also be used in planning meals.

CONSIDERATION OF PERSONAL NEEDS

Although we all have certain basic characteristics in common, each one of us has different dietary needs. Children, for example, need to eat differently than adults, while the needs of a person who is physically active differ from those of someone who is sedentary. We all have our own preferences when it comes to food. These and other individual differences need to be considered when choosing and preparing daily food.

In general, an optimum daily diet in a temperate, four-season climate consists of about 50-60 percent whole cereal grains; 5 percent (one or two small bowls) soup, preferably flavored with natural, high-quality seasonings such as miso or tamari soy sauce; 25-30 percent vegetables prepared in a variety of styles; and 5-10 percent beans and sea vegetables. Supplementary foods include occasional locally grown fruits, preferably cooked; white-meat fish; and a variety of seasonings, condiments, beverages, and natural snacks such as seeds and nuts. These suggestions are referred to as the standard macrobiotic diet, and are explained in more detail below and can serve as a general guide for creating a healthful diet in a temperate climate.

Personal health is also an important factor in determining the best way to interpret these guidelines. For example, a person in good overall health who adopts macrobiotics can interpret these guidelines more liberally, while someone who is ill needs to exercise greater care in the selection and preparation of daily food. Special modifications may also be necessary; for example, it may be appropriate to do things such as limit the intake of oil, raw salad, baked flour products, nuts, fruit, and other foods normally included in the standard macrobiotic diet. It may also be necessary to prepare a variety of special dishes or drinks to accelerate the discharge of fats or other forms of excess or to help strengthen particular organs. These

High-Quality Essentials

Our health depends on what we eat. It is important, therefore, to obtain essential nutrients from the highest quality sources. Guidelines are presented below:

Water. High-quality, clean, natural water is recommended for cooking and drinking. Spring or well water is fine for regular use, while chemically treated and distilled water are best avoided.

Carbohydrates. It is better to eat carbohydrates mostly in the form of polysaccharide glucose, a complex carbohydrate found in whole grains, vegetables (especially those with naturally sweet flavors), beans, sea vegetables, and chestnuts. Minimize or avoid the intake of simple sugars (mono- or disaccharides), such as those in fruit, honey, refined sugar, and other concentrated sweeteners.

Protein. It is better to obtain protein primarily from vegetable sources like whole grains, beans, and bean products, and to reduce reliance on animal proteins.

Fat. The hard, saturated fats found in most animal foods are best minimized or avoided. High-quality, unsaturated fats such as those in vegetable oils are better for regular use.

Salt. Natural sea salt contains a variety of trace minerals and is recommended for regular use. Refined salt, which is almost 100 percent sodium chloride with no trace minerals, is best avoided.

Vitamins and Minerals. It is better to obtain vitamins and minerals in their whole form as a part of natural foods rather than in isolated form as supplements.

adjustments are usually temporary, and the broader guidelines of the standard macrobiotic diet can normally be adopted once health is restored.

LIFESTYLE CHANGES

Together with eating well, there are a number of practices that complement a balanced natural diet and enhance the recovery of health. Keeping physically active, developing a positive outlook, and using natural cooking utensils, fabrics, and materials in the home are especially recommended. In the past, people lived more closely with nature and ate a more balanced natural diet. With each generation, we have gotten further from our roots in nature, and have experienced a corresponding increase in cancer and other chronic illnesses. These suggestions complement the macrobiotic diet and can help everyone enjoy more satisfying and harmonious living:

☐ Live each day happily without being preoccupied with your health; try to keep mentally and physically active.

☐ View everything and everyone you meet with gratitude; in particular, offer thinks before and after each meal.

☐ Please chew your food very well, at least fifty times per mouthful, or until it becomes liquid.

The complex carbohydrates in whole grains, beans, vegetables, and other whole natural foods are digested largely in the mouth through interaction with the enzymes in saliva. Chewing mixes food with saliva and facilitates smooth digestion and efficient absorption of nutrients. Chewing enables us to obtain more nutrients from less food. It also releases the medicinal properties of daily foods and is the key to improving, rather than simply maintaining, our state of health. Saliva is known to have antibacterial effects and, as reported in the May 1988 *Journal of the American Dental Association*, has been shown in laboratory experiments to prevent the AIDS virus from infecting white blood cells.

☐ It is best to avoid wearing synthetic or woolen clothes directly on the skin. Wear cotton as much as possible, especially for undergarments. Avoid excessive metallic accessories on the fingers, wrists, or neck. Keep such ornaments simple and graceful.

☐ To increase circulation, scrub your entire body with a hot, damp towel every morning or every night. If that is not possible, at least do your hands, fingers, feet, and toes.

☐ Initiate and maintain active correspondence, extending your best wishes to parents, children, brothers and sisters, teachers, and friends. Keep your personal relationships smooth and happy.

Exercise and Activity

For many of us, modern life offers fewer physically and mentally challenging circumstances than in the past. We are in danger of becoming a nation of "couch potatoes." Surveys have shown, for example, that a shockingly high percentage of American schoolchildren are overweight and unable to perform minimum tests of strength and endurance. These surveys also reveal that the average American family spends up to seven hours a day sitting in front of the television. A sedentary lifestyle causes stagnation of such bodily functions as the generation of caloric and electromagnetic energy, the circulation of blood and lymph, and the activity of the digestive and nervous systems. Physical activity is essential for good health; therefore, it is advisable to supplement the sedentary patterns of modern life with regular exercise. Below are suggestions for activating energy flow and reversing stagnation in body and mind:

Daily Body Scrubbing. Scrubbing your body with a moist, hot towel is a wonderful way to relieve stress, relax tension, and energize your life. It also activates circulation, softens deposits of hard fat below the skin, opens the pores, and allows excess to be actively discharged. For maximum effect, you can body scrub twice a day: once in the morning and again in the evening.

Body scrubbing can be done before or after a bath or shower, or anytime. All you need is a sink with hot water and a medium-sized cotton bath towel. Turn on the hot water. Hold the towel at either end and place the center of the towel under the stream of hot water. Wring out the towel, and while it is still hot and steamy, begin to scrub with it. Do one section of the body at a time. For example, begin with the hands and fingers and work your way up the arms to the shoulders, neck, and face, then down to the chest, upper back, abdomen, lower back, buttocks, legs, feet, and toes. Scrub until the skin becomes slightly red or until each part becomes warm. Reheat the towel by running it under hot water after scrubbing each section or as soon as the towel starts to cool.

A Daily Half-Hour Walk. A study published in the *Journal of the American Medical Association* in November 1989 concluded that moderate exercise, including a brisk half-hour walk every day, reduces the risk of cancer and heart disease. The researchers discovered that people who exercise moderately tend to live longer, and they added to the evidence that exercise can help prevent cancer, a relationship discovered only in the past several years. Scientists theorize that exercise increases bowel motility, a factor that helps prevent colon cancer. According to Carl Caspersen, an epidemiologist at the Center for Disease Control, "You don't have to be a marathoner to greatly reduce your mortality. After that first jump in activity, you're not buying that much more reduced risk."

Walking activates circulation, improves breathing, tones the muscles, and improves appetite. By increasing breathing capacity and activating circulation, walking helps cleanse the blood. The added oxygen in the blood oxidizes (burns) impurities, and the lymphatic system, which carries waste from the cells, also cleanses itself. Walking helps dissolve stress and tension too, and calms and clears the mind. We recommend taking a half-hour walk each day if your condition permits.

- ☐ Avoid taking long hot baths or showers unless you have been consuming too much salt or animal food.
- ☐ If your strength permits, walk on the beach, grass, or soil up to one-half hour every day; wear simple clothes. Keep your home in good order, from the kitchen, bathroom, and living rooms to every corner of the house.
- ☐ Avoid chemically perfumed cosmetics. To care for your teeth, brush with natural preparations or sea salt.
- ☐ In addition to taking a half-hour walk each day, include activities such as scrubbing floors, cleaning, washing clothes, and working in the yard or garden as part of your daily life. You may also participate in exercise programs such as yoga, martial arts, dance, or sports if your condition permits.
- ☐ Avoid using electric cooking devices (ovens and ranges) or microwave ovens. Convert to gas or wood-stove cooking at the earliest opportunity.
- ☐ It is best to minimize the use of color television and computer display terminals.

The health hazards of electromagnetic fields can no longer be ruled out, according to a July 1989 article in the science section of *The New York Times*. In addition to high voltage power lines, TVs, computers, and other electronic equipment, common household appliances such as vacuum cleaners, toasters, blenders, and fluorescent lights can be harmful to health. A background paper issued in 1989 by the Congressional Office of Technology Assessment stated, "It is now clear that low frequency electromagnetic fields can interact with individual cells and organs to produce biological changes." Laboratory experiments suggest that electromagnetic fields can interfere with DNA and stimulate chemicals in cells that are linked to cancer. Epidemiological studies have shown that women who used video display terminals for more than twenty hours a week in the first trimester of pregnancy suffered nearly twice as many miscarriages as women doing other types of office work. These studies also revealed that children who lived near electrical distribution lines were twice as likely to develop cancer as those who did not.

☐ Place large green plants in your house to freshen and enrich the oxygen content of the air in your home.

☐ Sing a happy song every day in order to activate your breathing and lift your spirits.

CREATING HEALTH

As we gain a better understanding of the way that diet and lifestyle influence health and sickness, we are in a better position to make healthful changes in our daily lives. We shift from a passive to an active role in creating health. The responsibility for making these changes is up to us. No one can take that responsibility for us. We are the ones who must initiate healthful changes and sustain them from day to day.

3

Diet and the
Development of Cancer

To better understand how diet influences cancer, we can refer to the image of a tree. A tree's structure is opposite to that of the human body. Body cells develop internally, while the leaves of a tree develop externally. A tree absorbs nutrients through external roots. The roots of the body are deep inside in the region of the small intestine where nutrients are absorbed. It is here that they enter the bloodstream and are distributed to the body's cells.

When a tree grows in healthy soil, it receives balanced nourishment and is able to thrive. But if the soil is deficient in minerals or contaminated with chemical toxins, the tree becomes unhealthy, and its leaves eventually wither and die. A naturally balanced diet is like healthy soil. When the body is properly nourished, the quality of the blood is sound, and the cells function in a normal way. If food becomes unbalanced, the quality of the blood begins to deteriorate, and the body's cells may eventually become unhealthy and even cancerous. The leaves of the tree depend on the nutrients absorbed through the roots. Similarly, the health of the cells depends on the quality of nutrients received by the body.

An unbalanced diet sets in motion a downward spiral of physical deterioration in which cancer is often the final, life-threatening stage. This process sometimes takes years to reach a critical point. Meanwhile, as this downward spiral gathers momentum, a variety of precancerous symptoms appear throughout the body. Although these symptoms seem unrelated to one another or to cancer, they are actually stages in an ongoing process that frequently culminates in the formation of a tumor. Cancer does not appear suddenly out of nowhere, but develops over time out of a chronically precancerous condition. To prevent cancer, we must reverse the direction of this spiral by changing our diet, lifestyle, and condition as a whole. Below we describe the stages in this process of change, beginning with a general description of balance or health.

HEALTHY EQUILIBRIUM

Health depends on our ability to maintain a condition of homeostasis—or dynamic equilibrium—in the body. Striking a balance between what we take in (in the form of food), and what we use for body repair and maintenance, and what we discharge in the form of energy and waste, is vitally important in maintaining optimal health. When we eat a well-balanced diet—both in terms of the quality of foods we eat and the quantities we take in—we provide the body with what it needs, and our day-to-day functions of elimination—urination, bowel movement, breathing, perspiration—are sufficient to discharge any excess and to keep us in good health.

Physical activity helps keep the body free of toxic accumulation; this is why regular exercise helps reduce the risk of degenerative disease. No wonder a traditional people such as the Hunza, who eat a moderately balanced diet while maintaining a vigorous rural lifestyle, have remained cancer-free.

Women have several additional biological functions that help them discharge excess. The monthly menstrual cycle helps a woman to discharge more efficiently, as do having children and breast-feeding. Breast-feeding allows a portion of the excess that builds up in a woman's body during pregnancy to be discharged, thus protecting her from potentially harmful accumulations. This is one reason that researchers have noted a negative correlation between breast-feeding and the development of breast cancer. Men often need to compensate for the lack of such built-in discharge mechanisms by being more physically active.

ABNORMAL DISCHARGES

Because the modern diet is so unbalanced, most people take in more than they are able to healthfully discharge. This disturbs the body's equilibrium, and, in order to restore balance, a variety of abnormal discharge mechanisms are set in motion. Abnormal discharges can be acute or chronic; they can start early or late in life. In their initial stages, discharges tend to be self-limiting, which means that their symptoms normally disappear once the excess has been eliminated from the body. However, if the underlying dietary causes are not changed, the discharges may become chronic or recurring.

Chronic discharges often begin in infancy, primarily because of the modern habit of feeding babies cow's milk formulas rather than breast milk. The balance of nutrients in breast milk matches the needs of the baby, while cow's milk contains an excessive amount of saturated fat, protein, and minerals that tax the body's digestive and excretory systems. If the body's normal channels of discharge are overwhelmed, a variety of abnormal discharge symptoms occur to get rid of the excess—diarrhea, digestive upsets, chest congestion, and skin rashes. These conditions are more common in bottle-fed babies than in breast-fed babies, and often persist into adulthood, especially when plenty of dairy and other animal products and simple sugars continue being consumed.

Casein, the primary protein in cow's milk, is relatively insoluble in the digestive tract of a human infant. It is utilized with only about 50 percent efficiency. The remaining protein is unused and becomes excess that must be discharged. Some passes through the digestive tract and is discharged in the feces, while some is digested but cannot be utilized by the cells and is excreted in the urine. The excess protein, mineral salts, and saturated fat in cow's milk can easily overwhelm the body's capacities for discharge—both normal and abnormal—and will then accumulate internally, setting the stage for the next step in the spiral of declining health.

Similarly, the excessive amounts of protein, fat, sugar, and chemical additives in the modern diet as a whole also disturb the body's equilibrium. Recurring conditions such as inner ear infections, sore throats, colds and flu, and tonsillitis are common in the modern world, and are indicative of the excessive nature of modern eating patterns. Although symptoms such as these can be unpleasant, they actually have a beneficial purpose, as they represent the body's attempt to get rid of excess and restore equilibrium. Allergies, for example, represent the body's attempt to discharge excessive factors through the nasal and respiratory passages or through the skin. Allergic reactions actually help the body eliminate excess and slow the rate of toxic accumulation. As a result, people who suffer from allergies are statistically less prone to develop cancer, which, as we will see, is promoted by the chronic accumulation of excess in the body.

Unfortunately, most people today don't realize that symptoms such as these may also be a direct result of what they have been eating. The common perception is that they are caused by some outside factor such as cold viruses, streptococcus bacteria, or pollen. Rather than tolerating the discharge and changing the dietary imbalances that have caused it, people usually try to suppress the symptoms with medication. Of course, in serious or life-threatening situations, this may be necessary, but it is important to remember that medications do not solve the underlying problem and often weaken the body's ability to discharge. As a result, some of the excess that would normally be eliminated remains in the body where it can contribute to a more serious condition in the future.

Skin diseases are another form of chronic discharge. The repeated intake of excess, stresses and eventually weakens the kidneys and intestines. These organs are forced to work overtime in order to cope with the overload of protein, fat, sugar, and toxic chemicals contained in an unbalanced diet. When these organs cannot handle the overload, excess is discharged through the skin, which results in skin markings, growths, and discolorations, or skin diseases such as eczema or acne. Freckles and aging spots, for example, are caused by the discharge of refined and other simple sugars. White patches show that milk, cottage cheese, and other dairy products are being discharged, while warts, moles, and excess body hair are produced by the

Macrobiotic Miracles

MARLENE MCKENNA

In 1983 Marlene McKenna was diagnosed with malignant melanoma. "As a working mother of four children, radio and TV commentator, and investment broker, I was living a very unbalanced life," Marlene explained in an interview in *The Providence Journal.*

In August 1985, she began to complain of severe stomach pains, and in January 1986, doctors discovered that five tumors had spread throughout her body. Two feet of her intestines were removed, and Marlene was told she had six months to a year to live.

Declining all treatments, Marlene turned to macrobiotics at the suggestion of her brother and visited Michio Kushi in Boston. In addition to changing her diet, she replaced her electric stove with a gas stove, and began to meditate and practice yoga. A devout Catholic, she also did a lot of inspirational reading and praying.

"I promised God that if He walked me through this and helped me live, I would give Him life with life," she recalls.

Within a year she was on the way to recovery, and doctors found no evidence of further cancer. Feeling well enough to return to public life, she ran for state treasurer in Rhode Island. During the campaign, she discovered that she was pregnant. Because of her previous illness and age (forty-two), doctors encouraged her to have an abortion. Marlene refused. "I realized that (having the baby) was part of my promise to give life with life," she explains. Though she lost the election, she gave birth to a healthy baby boy, keeping her promise to God and proving her physicians wrong.

Since then, she has opened Shepherd's, a macrobiotic natural foods restaurant in Providence, and is helping people around the country who have heard of her remarkable recovery.

VIRGINIA BROWN

In August 1978, Virginia Brown, a fifty-six-year-old mother and registered nurse from Tunbridge, Vermont, noticed a black mole on her arm that kept getting bigger and blacker. She had lost a lot of weight and felt very dull mentally. Doctors at Vermont Medical Center in Burlington performed a biopsy and discovered that she had an advanced case of malignant melanoma (Stage

IV). The physicians told her that without surgery she could expect to live only six months. "Even though I had been trained and had practiced in the medical profession for years," Virginia later recalled, "I could not go along with surgery. I had professed alternatives for years, but did not really practice them."

At home, her son and daughter-in-law encouraged her to try macrobiotics, and shortly thereafter she attended the East West Foundation's annual cancer conference, meeting that year in Amherst, Massachusetts. At the conference she listened to fifteen cancer patients discuss their experiences with the diet and was impressed with their accounts.

Prior to that time, Virginia had followed the standard American way of eating, high in refined foods and fat, especially animal fat from dairy foods, beef, poultry, and fish. At the time she started the diet, she was so sick that she could hardly make it upstairs and slept most of the day. After three weeks of eating the new food, which her children prepared for her, she experienced a change in her energy level, attitude, and mental clarity. "I was a new person, I could get up and walk around."

In September, Virginia went to Boston to see Michio Kushi, and he made more specific dietary recommendations and advised her to study cooking. With the support of her family, she adhered faithfully to the diet, supplemented by yoga, prayer and meditation, and a two-mile walk each morning after breakfast.

In 1979, it became apparent that Virginia had overcome her condition, and medical exams subsequently confirmed her recovery. After restoring her health, Virginia went on to study at the Kushi Institute and to work as a nurse in the macrobiotic health program that was started at the Lemuel Shattuck Hospital in Boston, promoting a more natural way of living among other medical professionals and patients. In 1984, her story was published by Japan Publications in the book *Macrobiotic Miracle: How a Vermont Family Overcame Cancer*.

BETTY METZGER

During the month of August 1980, Betty Metzger underwent surgery for malignant melanoma. That consisted of removing an area of tissue about 4½-inches in diameter down to the muscle on her right shoulder. Skin was grafted from her thigh. The surgery healed nicely and after a few months she felt reasonably secure that her cancer problem was solved.

However, in November 1981 there appeared a lump on the right side of Betty's neck. The cancer had spread to the lymph nodes. Betty's surgeon removed the cancerous nodes and during the week before Christmas 1981, she received chemotherapy for five consecutive days. There would be a three-week rest before the next regimen of five daily treatments. Betty's oncologist said this would continue for a year at which time they would reevaluate her condition.

Chemotherapy was halted from the first of June to the end of August because of low white blood cell counts. Betty received the August treatments and three days of the September regimen when she felt that she could no longer go on.

A friend told Betty about Dr. Sattilaro's account of his surviving cancer in the August [1982] issue of *Life*. She and her husband read *Recalled by Life* by Dr. Sattilaro and Jean and Mary Alice Kohler's book *Healing Miracles from Macrobiotics*. That and her family's encouragement were all Betty needed to embark on a macrobiotic way of life. She sought and found much help from friends who were on the diet and read everything about it that was available.

"It has now been nine years since my first cancer surgery," says Betty. "I feel great, thanking God every day for the precious gift of good health."

Sources: One Peaceful World, Autumn, 1989; *Malignant Melanoma, Stage IV, Cancer and Diet* (East West Foundation, 1980); interview with Alex Jack, September 30, 1982; *Macrobiotic Miracle: How a Vermont Family Overcame Cancer* (Japan Publications, 1984); correspondence with Betty Metzger, Shelby, Ohio, August 16, 1989.

overconsumption of protein and fats. Skin cancer—the most common form of cancer in the United States—also represents the chronic discharge of dietary excess.

Colds and flu enable the body to discharge dietary excess. The symptoms of a cold are usually nasal discharge—including a runny nose—sneezing, coughing, and fever. Pink, watery eyes, and a whitish-yellow eye discharge sometimes accompany colds, as do irregular bowel movements and diarrhea.

Colds primarily involve the upper respiratory organs—the throat, sinuses, and nasal passages. The flu also affects these areas, but usually produces more generalized symptoms throughout the body. In some cases, it involves the digestive organs, a condition commonly referred to as intestinal flu.

When the discharge of a cold involves the upper body—for example, the nasal passages, head, and throat—the primary cause is the excessive intake of extremely expansive foods or beverages such as simple sugars, concentrated sweeteners, fruit and fruit juice, spices, soft drinks, and ice cream. When the discharge affects the lungs and organs in the mid-section, including the stomach, the primary cause is the excessive intake of fats and oils in addition to the expansive foods. Discharges that affect the intestines and organs in the lower body are triggered by the excessive intake of more densely saturated animal fats in addition to the items mentioned previously.

The key to preventing colds and flu lies in avoiding the extremes in diet that lead to recurring discharges. A macrobiotic diet helps unblock the body's normal discharge pathways, and thus strengthens natural resistance. When a cold occurs, the best course of action is to rest and eat simply, and let it run its course. Moreover, natural home care preparations such as those presented in *The Macrobiotic Cancer Prevention Cookbook* can help ease the symptoms of a cold without interfering with the process of discharge.

THE BUILDUP OF EXCESS

Continual overindulgence in fat, sugar, protein, and chemical additives overburdens and can eventually overwhelm the body's ability to discharge. Excess then begins to accumulate throughout the body in the form of deposits of mucus and fat. This process is particularly problematic when the skin becomes hard and inelastic and when its ability to discharge diminishes. Overconsumption of saturated fat and cholesterol is a major cause of this condition.

The skin is richly supplied with blood vessels. When saturated fat and cholesterol accumulate in the capillaries that nourish the skin, the skin receives less blood, as well as less oxygen and nutrients. Cells depend on oxygen and nutrients for life, and if the supply of these vital factors diminishes, cells take longer to renew themselves. The speed at which new skin cells form in the lowest layer of the epidermis and migrate out to the surface of the body decreases. A dull, flaky film then develops on the surface of the body as dead, dehydrated cells accumulate.

The construction of capillaries also reduces the skin's ability to remove waste products, resulting in an overall condition of accumulation and stagnation. Saturated fats accumulate in the sebaceous glands and sweat ducts in a similar way, and block the secretion of moisture and natural oils. The surface of the skin, therefore, does no receive enough moisture, and becomes hard and dry. This tight, constricted condition also interferes with elimination. To remedy this problem, reduce the intake of saturated fat and cholesterol, and practice the daily body-scrubbing routine outlined in Chapter 2.

At this stage, excess begins to accumulate inside the body, initially in the form of hard fat and mucous deposits. At first, these deposits form in parts of the body that interact with the outside, such as the sinuses, breasts, and reproductive tract. Deposits of fat and mucus commonly appear in the regions such as the sinuses and inner ear, which are discussed in greater detail on the pages that follow (see Figure 3.1).

Sinuses

The sinuses are a common site of mucus accumulation. Symptoms such as nasal congestion and sinusitis (inflammation of the sinuses) result from the underlying accumulation of mucus, as do hay fever and other allergies. Sometimes these deposits become so chronically severe that calcified stones start to form. Chronic sinusitis also produces headaches.

Mucus in the sinuses results primarily from the overconsumption of fatty and oily foods, including milk, ice cream, and other dairy products, and an excessive intake of simple sugars, including refined sugar, honey, maple syrup, concentrated sweeteners, chocolate, and fruits. Too much fluid or too many watery foods (such as raw fruits) also promote nasal blockage by causing the tissues in the sinuses and nasal passages to become swollen.

Inner Ear

The accumulation of mucus and fat in the inner ear interferes with the functioning of the hearing mechanism and can

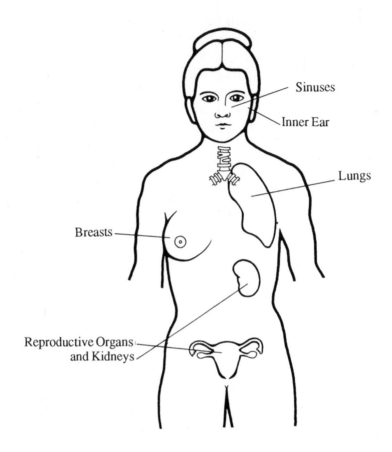

Figure 3.1   Sites of Mucus and Fat Accumulation

lead to pain, infection, impaired hearing, and even deafness. About twelve million Americans are now deaf, and millions more suffer from various degrees of hearing impairment.

Ear infections result when the accumulation of excess fosters the growth of viruses or bacteria, and when natural immunity is weakened by the overconsumption of sugar, tropical fruits, drugs and medications, and fatty animal foods. The most common site of ear infection is the region behind the eardrum. Infection here is called *otitis media*, or middle ear infection. Pain frequently results when accumulated excess— including fluid, mucus, or infection—hampers the normal drainage of the ear through the Eustachian tubes. Recurrent middle ear infections are quite common today, especially among children. Tympanostomy, or the surgical puncturing of the eardrum to allow drainage of fluid, has surpassed ton-sillectomy as the most common surgery among children.

The ears are also sensitive to cold or iced foods or beverages. The overconsumption of ice cream, soft drinks, and other chilled or iced foods is a frequent cause of inner ear problems.

Lungs

The lungs are another common site for the accumulation of mucus and fats. Symptoms like coughing, chest congestion, and chronic bronchitis often result from these accumulations. Mucus may also accumulate in the alveoli, or minute air sacs deep in the lungs, and deposits of saturated fat may start to clog the capillaries that surround the sacs. These conditions reduce the amount of oxygen absorbed by the bloodstream, and slow the discharge of carbon dioxide, thus increasing the concentration of toxins in the blood.

Mucus in the bronchi can be dislodged by coughing, but once it accumulates in the air sacs, it becomes more firmly lodged and can remain there for years. Then, if air pollutants or cigarette smoke enter the lungs, their heavier components are attracted to and remain in this sticky environment. Over time, these irritants can combine with dietary excess to promote the development of cancer. However, underlying the process of carcinogenesis is the chronic accumulation of fat and mucus in the alveoli and capillaries that surround them. Lung cancer is one of the leading killers in the United States today. About 157,000 new cases of lung cancer are diagnosed in this country each year.

Breasts

The accumulation of mucus and fat in the breasts often causes hardening and thickening of the breast tissue. In many cases, it leads to fibrocystic disease. Excess usually accumulates here in the form of mucus and deposits of fatty acid, both of which take the form of a thick, heavy liquid. These deposits harden into cysts when cheese, poultry, and other hard animal fats are eaten excessively. In the presence of these foods, the deposits may consolidate and promote the development of hard breast tumors. Foods like ice cream, milk, chocolate, and sugar cause the deposits to assume a softer, more liquid form (less consolidation). When eaten excessively, they promote the development of soft breast tumors. Breast cancer currently affects one in ten American women, and is increasing in incidence. About 150,000 new cases of breast cancer are diagnosed each year in the United States. Figure 3.2 shows the relationship between dietary fat and cancer worldwide.

In the *Cancer Prevention Diet* we cite numerous studies that have shown a positive correlation between the consumption of animal fat and the incidence of breast cancer. (Obesity and consumption of refined sugar have also been linked to this disease.) Several newer studies have appeared since the *Cancer Prevention Diet* was published in 1983. A report in the February 15, 1989, issue of the *Journal of the National Cancer Institute* described a study on diet and breast cancer conducted in Vercelli, a province in northwestern Italy. The Vercelli study confirmed the link between fats and/or calories

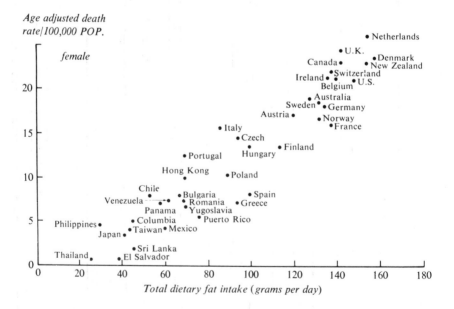

Figure 3.2   Relationship Between Breast Cancer and Dietary
Fat Intake

and breast cancer, and implicated saturated fats and animal proteins as the most potent risk factors.

In this study, Paolo Toniolo, an epidemiologist at New York University Medical Center, compared the diets of 250 women with breast cancer with those of 499 healthy women of the same age. Carbohydrate consumption between the two groups was found to be generally the same, while a higher protein and fat intake was noted in the breast cancer group, due primarily to a higher intake of meat and dairy products. A report on the study in *Science News* noted, ". . . the biggest difference between the two groups was that women with breast cancer tended to consume considerably more milk, high-fat cheese, and butter."

Commenting on the breast cancer and diet connection, Maureen Henderson, an epidemiologist at the Fred Hutchenson Cancer Research Center in Seattle, told *Time* (January 1991), "I'm sure of it. The results are too consistent to believe that the association is indirect." Japan has traditionally had a low rate of breast cancer. However, this is now changing—the rate of breast cancer in Japan increased 58 percent between 1975 and 1985. Dr. Akira Eboshida of the Ministry of Health and Welfare in Japan attributes the increase to recent changes in the Japanese diet. He stated in *Time*, "The largest factor behind the sharp rise is the Westernization of eating habits. We are eating more animal fat and less fiber."

Reproductive Organs

The prostate gland is a common site for the accumulation of mucus and fat. Often, the first stages of trouble in the prostate are microscopic nodules, known as prostatic concretions, that appear in the alkaline fluid secreted by the gland. If plenty of hard fats are consumed, especially the kinds in meat, eggs, cheese, and poultry, the concretions may harden and calcify. Prostatic concretions often accumulate as cysts in the tissue of the gland.

As additional fats accumulate, the prostate begins to enlarge. Benign prostatic enlargement has become nearly universal among modern men: it is estimated that 10 percent experience it by the age of 40 and practically 100 percent by the age of 60. The end result of this process of accumulation is often prostate cancer, a condition that currently affects about 106,000 men per year in the United States.

The female reproductive organs are also a common site for the buildup of fat and mucus. Fibroids, or fleshy growths in the uterus, are common today and result from the accumulation of fats in the muscle of the uterus. Fibroids often begin as small seedlings. Whether or not they enlarge depends on the quality and volume of fat and other forms of excess eaten by the woman. Frequently, they continue growing as the result of an improper diet. Fibroids may grow to become quite large, even to the size of a football, and may begin to cause pain as a result of pressing on other organs.

In the extreme, these accumulations can promote the cell changes that lead to cancer. There are an estimated 46,500 new cases of uterine cancer each year in the United States. Approximately 33,000 of these cancers are found in the body of the uterus (most often in the endometrium, or lining of the uterus); about 13,500 cases are cervical cancer.

The process whereby ovarian cysts and tumors develop is similar to that in which fibroids are created. There are dozens of varieties of ovarian growths, and each is the result of a specific excess in the woman's diet. Ovarian cancer, the end result of the accumulation of excess in the ovaries, especially of the hard fats in eggs, cheese, poultry, and meat, annually affects about 20,500 women in the United States.

Excess fat and mucus in the female reproductive tract is frequently expelled through the vagina, producing a variety of vaginal discharges. The localization of excess in this region disturbs the normal acidity of the vagina, providing a medium for the growth of various organisms that promote infection.

Among natural home remedies, a sea salt hip bath and bancha tea douche can help reduce the buildup of fat and mucus in the female reproductive tract. To prepare this traditional remedy, place a large, double handful of sea salt in hot bath water. Fill the tub with enough water to cover your navel, and sit in the hot bath water for about ten minutes. Cover your upper body with a dry towel to keep from becoming chilled. After soaking your lower body for ten minutes, prepare a special douching solution with warm bancha tea, a three-finger pinch of sea salt, and the juice from half a lemon. Use the solution immediately after the hip bath. This traditional remedy is especially effective when done twice a week for about a month, during which time it is important to avoid extremes and to eat a clean, naturally balanced diet.

Kidneys and Bladder

Deposits of mucus and fat also accumulate in the kidneys, clogging the minute tubules, or nephrons, that filter the blood. The buildup of fats in these tissues accelerates the formation of insoluble waste—such as kidney stones—and the gradual loss of nephrons. A healthy young person has about a million nephrons, but after age thirty, the number starts to decline. As a person ages, the number may decline by as much as a third. The consumption of saturated fat and cholesterol causes a gradual thickening and stiffening of the arteries that supply the kidneys with blood. This can lead to constriction of the capillaries that are interwoven with the nephrons, and through which waste products are discharged from the blood. These degenerative changes interfere with the filtration of the blood and contribute to the buildup of toxins in the bloodstream.

The accumulation of fat and mucus in the bladder often leads to frequent bladder infections and to the formation of bladder stones. In extreme cases, these accumulations promote cell changes and cancer. There are currently 49,000 new cases of bladder cancer per year in the United States. Cancer of the bladder is the fifth most common cancer among American men and the ninth most common cancer among women.

FURTHER DETERIORATION

In many cases, the preceding regions can no longer absorb excess, and deposits of fat and mucus start to form in other internal organs. One example is the accumulation of cholesterol and saturated fat in the arteries and blood vessels that supply

Monitoring Internal Accumulations

Accumulations of fat and mucus can be monitored by observing markings and discolorations in the whites of the eyes. The following figure shows several of these correlations:

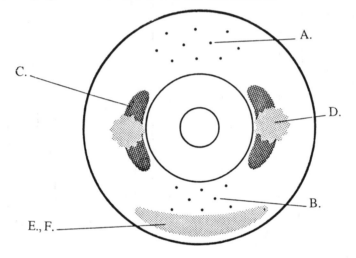

Figure 3.3   Markings and Discolorations in the Whites of the Eyes.

A. Tiny dark spots in the top of the white of the eye frequently indicate the formation of calcified deposits in the sinuses.

B. Dark spots in the bottom of the white of the eye often indicate the formation of kidney stones. Ovarian cysts may also be indicated.

C., D. The accumulation of mucus and fat in the liver, gallbladder, spleen, and pancreas frequently appears as a blue, green, or brownish shade, or as white patches in the middle of the eye on either side of the iris.

E. Accumulation of fat and mucus in and around the prostate is often indicated by a yellowish discoloration in the lower part of the eyeball.

F. Fat and mucus in the female sex organs are also indicated by the yellowish discoloration in E, above. Vaginal discharges, ovarian cysts, fibroid tumors, and other gynecological disorders are possibly indicated.

the heart. Narrowing or blocking of these blood vessels is quite common today due to the modern high-fat diet and is a leading cause of angina pains and heart attack.

The pancreas is another common site for the accumulation of fat, especially the type of fat found in chicken, cheese, and eggs. These accumulations interfere with the secretion of pancreatic hormones, most often glucagon, or anti-insulin. Insulin and anti-insulin work in a complementary way to regulate the level of glucose, or sugar, in the blood. Insulin causes the blood sugar level to go down, while anti-insulin causes it to rise. The accumulation of fats in the pancreas causes the organ to become hard and tight, and frequently leads to a deficiency of anti-insulin. The result is a condition of chronic low blood sugar, or hypoglycemia, and an almost constant craving for sugar, soft drinks, chocolate, alcohol, and other foods or drinks that cause the blood sugar to rapidly rise.

In the extreme, the chronic buildup of fats in the pancreas promotes the development of cancer. Worldwide, the rate of pancreatic cancer is higher in countries where a large volume of animal fats is consumed. The death rate for pancreatic cancer has also been rising in the United States, increasing 24 percent among men and 32 percent among women from 1950–1985. Currently, about 28,100 new cases are diagnosed each year in the United States.

Fat and mucus also accumulate in the liver and gallbladder, creating the background for conditions such as hepatitis and gallstones. They also accumulate in and around the bones, muscles, and lymphatic system, as well as in the brain. In each of these areas, the accumulation of fats and other toxic substances can promote the development of cancer. A critical stage in this process is reached when the internal organs contain deposits of mucus and fat, and when discharge through the kidneys, intestines, lungs, and skin is severely hampered by these deposits. This condition produces toxicity in the blood and promotes the development of cancer.

As long as a person continues eating saturated fats, refined sugar, excess protein, chemical additives, and other potential cancer-promoting substances, the body will continue to deposit toxins in the area of the tumor. Not only do many of these substances feed the tumor, they also inhibit the immune system's ability to neutralize and discharge cancer cells and other toxins. When the original site of the tumor can no longer absorb excess, the body begins depositing toxins in another location, and as a result, the cancer spreads. Unless there is a change in eating habits, the disease will continuously grow and spread as a matter of course.

When cancer develops, a greenish color will often appear on the skin. This color reflects the process of cell deterioration that is occurring inside the body. Red is the color of the animal kingdom, and is apparent in the color of the blood. Vegetables and other forms of plant life are based on green chlorophyll. Eating represents the process whereby we transform green vegetable life into red blood. Cancer represents a reverse process in which body cells begin changing back to a more primitive form. This process frequently manifests as a greenish shade appearing on the surface of the body. Samples of this may be seen in Figure 3.4.

Discoloration usually appears along the meridians, or pathways of energy that run near the surface of the body. These invisible channels conduct electromagnetic energy to and from the body's organs and functions. Breast cancer, for example, often appears as a thin green line that begins at the wrist and extends up the center of the inner forearm. This discoloration corresponds to the heart governor meridian and mirrors the condition of the upper chest. In the case of colon cancer, a greenish color often appears on the region of the large intestine meridian located on the outside of either hand in the indented area between the thumb and forefinger. Additional correlations are presented in Table 3.1.

A greenish discoloration may also appear before a tumor has started to develop, and indicates that a precancerous condition is developing in the corresponding organ. When someone with a precancerous discoloration begins to eat a naturally balanced diet, this greenish shade often disappears, an indication that the precancerous condition has been reversed.

As we can see, symptoms such as vaginal discharges, breast and ovarian cysts, skin diseases, dry skin, hypoglycemia, and fibroids are actually precancerous conditions. However, this process need not reach its conclusion in cancer. The progressive development of cancer can be halted and reversed through a change in diet and lifestyle, while many of the

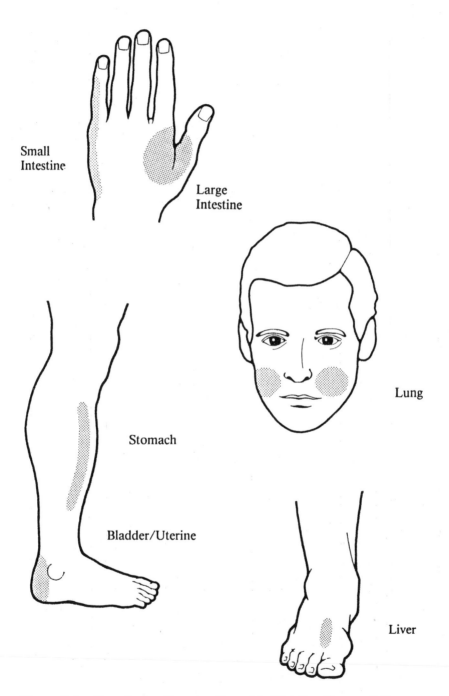

Figure 3.4   Correlation Between Greenish Discolorations and Cancer

Table 3.1   Correlations Between Discolorations and Cancer Sites

Cancer Type	Region Where Greenish Shade Might Appear
Small Intestine	Outside of the little finger.
Lung	Either or both cheeks.
Stomach	Along the outside front of either leg, especially below the knee.
Bladder/Uterine	Around either ankle on the outside of the leg.
Liver	Around the top of the foot in the central area.

symptoms of accumulation and discharge can be relieved by the use of macrobiotic home health care remedies such as those presented in the *Macrobiotic Cancer Prevention Cookbook*. Managing our condition through diet and non-toxic, natural methods of home care is the essence of the macrobiotic approach.

In the chapter that follows, we take a closer look at how the macrobiotic diet is in accord with the latest thinking about preventive nutrition, especially with the recommendations for reducing cancer risk made by leading public health agencies. Around the world, a consensus is building that diet is a primary factor influencing whether or not we are able to remain cancer-free.

4

Macrobiotics and Preventive Nutrition

In general, the macrobiotic diet is a healthful way of eating.

American Medical Association
Family Medical Guide

The typical modern diet overemphasizes the intake of fat (and, to a certain extent, protein), compromising the intake of complex carbohydrates and fiber. By one estimate, this dietary pattern means that 42 percent of our caloric intake is consumed as fat. Carbohydrates account for 46 percent—almost half of this is sugar—with the balance consumed as refined flour and cereal products, and canned or frozen fruits and vegetables. Lastly, the source of almost two-thirds of the protein intake on this diet is animal.

This diet is not based on sound principles of nutritional science, nor is it based upon the coevolution and biological codependence of the plant and animal kingdoms. Rather, it is a product of economic forces over the past two or three centuries.

More than at any other time in history, the health costs for persons consuming this diet are astronomical. Worldwide, these costs can currently be measured in billions of dollars and hundreds of thousands of lives every year. Obesity, heart disease, cancer, diabetes, hypertension, and a myriad of other degenerative illnesses can also be attributed to this dietary pattern, which is followed by the vast majority of people in the United States and other industrialized countries in both the East and West. Further, emerging Third World nations are, unfortunately, embracing modern dietary habits with the recent introduction of fast foods in Asia and the importation of baby formulas and other highly processed foods to South American and African nations.

Suggestions for a change of direction, as well as an outline of the health costs of the dietary pattern described above, are presented in the document *Dietary Goals for the United States* published in 1977 by the Select Committee on Nutrition and Human Needs of the United States Senate. These suggestions have been reiterated and supported by a number of other publications, including the National Academy of Sciences' report *Diet, Nutrition and Cancer*, published in June 1982, as well as in reports issued by the world's leading public health agencies over the past ten years.

These agencies have expressed the growing awareness of the preventive value of a diet based on whole grains, beans, fresh local vegetables, and other low-fat, high-fiber foods. Their guidelines point in the direction of the standard macrobiotic diet and have included the following:

- [ ] The United States Congress Senate Select Committee on Nutrition and Human Needs report, *Dietary Goals for the United States* (1976–1977).
- [ ] The United States Surgeon General's report, *Healthy People: Health Promotion and Disease Prevention* (1979).
- [ ] Dietary guidelines issued by the American Heart Association, the American Diabetes Association, the American Society for Clinical Nutrition, and the United States Department of Agriculture.
- [ ] A 1981 report by a panel of the American Association for the Advancement of Science.
- [ ] Interim dietary guidelines for preventing cancer issued by the National Academy of Sciences in the 1982 publication *Diet, Nutrition and Cancer*.

☐ Dietary guidelines issued by the National Cancer Institute and the American Cancer Society.

☐ Dietary guidelines in *The Surgeon General's Report on Nutrition and Health* (1988).

☐ Dietary guidelines in the National Academy of Sciences' report *Diet and Health* (1989).

The guidelines referred to as "the standard macrobiotic diet" are based, in good part, on traditional eating patterns, and it is increasingly clear that their introduction anticipated the scientific findings reported in the publications mentioned above. The standard macrobiotic diet may, therefore, hold the greatest potential for preventing the degenerative diseases plaguing us today.

The suggestions for dietary change in *Dietary Goals for the United States* and *Diet, Nutrition and Cancer* as well as in subsequent publications strikingly point to the possibilities in the standard macrobiotic diet. The macrobiotic diet can serve as a practical guide for changing the eating patterns of people in the United States and other industrialized countries.

In looking at these suggestions, remember that they are aimed at people who eat the standard American diet. This diet is characterized by high animal-food and sugar consumption, low consumption of cereal grains, and an abundance of highly processed and refined foods.

DIETARY GOALS FOR THE UNITED STATES

In 1977, the United States Senate Select Committee on Nutrition and Human Needs issued *Dietary Goals for the United States*, a landmark report on the nation's way of eating, its health, and future direction. Also known as the "McGovern Report" after its chairman, George McGovern, *Dietary Goals* concluded:

> During this century, the composition of the average diet in the United States has changed radically. Complex carbohydrates—fruit, vegetables, and grain products—which were the mainstay of the diet, now play a minority role. At the same time, fat and sugar consumption have

risen to the point where these two dietary elements alone now comprise at least 60 percent of the total calorie intake, up from 50 percent in the early 1900s.

In the view of doctors and nutritionists consulted by the Select Committee, these and other changes in the diet amount to a wave of malnutrition—both over- and under-consumption—that may be as profoundly damaging to the Nation's health as the widespread contagious diseases of the early part of this century. The over-consumption of fat, generally, and saturated fat in particular, as well as cholesterol, sugar, salt, and alcohol have been related to six of the leading causes of death: Heart disease, cancer, cerebrovascular diseases, diabetes, arteriosclerosis, and cirrhosis of the liver.

Dietary Goals went on to list seven suggestions, essentially advising increased consumption of complex carbohydrates and fiber, along with decreased consumption of sugar, fats, and salt:

1. Increase consumption of fruits and vegetables and whole grains.
2. Decrease consumption of refined and other processed sugars and foods high in such sugars.
3. Decrease consumption of foods high in total fat; in particular, replace saturated fats, whether obtained from animal or vegetable sources, with polyunsaturated fats.
4. Decrease consumption of animal fat, and choose meats, poultry, and fish that will reduce saturated fat intake.
5. Except for young children, substitute low-fat and non-fat milk for whole milk, and low-fat dairy products for high-fat dairy products.
6. Decrease consumption of butterfat, eggs, and other high cholesterol foods.
7. Decrease consumption of salt and foods high in salt.

The standard macrobiotic diet embodies practically every one of these points. Since the standard macrobiotic diet is centered around whole cereal grains and vegetables, the first suggestion is satisfied. Secondly, there is virtually no consumption of refined or processed sugars in the macrobiotic diet. "Sugars" come instead from the consumption of vegetables, fruit, and the occasional use of concentrated syrups made from whole grains.

Foods that are high in fat include animal foods such as beef, dairy food, and pork, none of which is customarily eaten on the macrobiotic diet, thereby satisfying suggestion number three. The primary sources of fat in the standard macrobiotic diet are whole grains and beans, and vegetable oils such as sesame and corn used in sautéing. These fat sources are predominately polyunsaturated, and their normal use results in considerably lower consumption of saturated fat than found in a typical American diet.

When animal food is consumed on the macrobiotic diet, the preferred form is _fish_, which generally contains less fat, especially saturated fat, than other animal foods (suggestion number four). The standard macrobiotic diet generally has little animal food—the sole source of dietary cholesterol—and is, consequently, very low in cholesterol, implementing suggestion number six.

GUIDELINES IN DIET, NUTRITION, AND CANCER

In 1982 the National Academy of Sciences issued *Diet, Nutrition and Cancer*, a 472-page report to the National Cancer Institute, in which the modern diet was associated with a majority of common cancers, especially malignancies of the stomach, colon, breast, endometrium, and lung. The panel reviewed hundreds of current medical studies associating long-term eating patterns with the incidence of cancer, and estimated that diet is responsible for 30 to 40 percent of cancers in men and 60 percent of cancers in women. The following are a few excerpts from the Academy's publication:

☐ "Just as it was once difficult for investigators to recognize that a symptom complex could be caused by the lack of a nutrient, so until recently has it been difficult for scientists to recognize that certain pathological conditions might result from an abundant and apparently normal diet. . . ."

☐ "Technological advances in recent years have led to changes in the methods of food processing, a greater as-

sortment of food products, and, as a result, changes in
the consumption patterns of the U.S. population. The
impact of these modifications on human health, especially the potential adverse effects of food additives and
contaminants, has drawn considerable attention from
the news media and the public. Advances in technology
have resulted in increased use of industrial chemicals,
thereby increasing the potential for chemical contamination of drinking water and food supplies. The use of processed foods, and, consequently, of additives, has also increased substantially during the past four decades. . . .
More than 55 percent of the food consumed in the
United States today has been processed to some degree
before distribution to the consumer . . ."

☐ "There is sufficient evidence that high fat consumption is
linked to increased incidence of certain cancers (notably
breast and colon cancer) and that low fat is associated
with a lower incidence of these cancers. The committee
recommends that the consumption of both saturated and
unsaturated fats be reduced in the average U.S. diet. An
appropriate and practical target is to reduce the intake
of fat from its present level (approximately 40 percent) to
30 percent of total calories in the diet. The scientific
data do not provide a strong basis for establishing fat intake at precisely 30 percent of total calories. Indeed, the
data could be used to justify an even greater reduction."

☐ "The committee emphasizes the importance of including
fruits, vegetables, and whole grain cereal products in the
daily diet. In epidemiological studies, frequent consumption of these foods has been inversely correlated with the
incidence of various cancers."

These and other recommendations in *Diet, Nutrition and
Cancer* point in the general direction of the standard macrobiotic diet. A brief summary of the Interim Dietary Guidelines set forth in this publication, "consistent with good nutrition and likely to reduce the risk of cancer," follows:

☐ The consumption of both saturated and unsaturated fats
should be reduced in the average American diet.
☐ It is important to include fruits, vegetables, and whole

grains in the daily diet. Various components of these foods, including some vitamins and other substances, have been shown to be of potential benefit in the prevention of cancer. However, the importance of these components does not justify the use of supplements to increase their intake. Because of the unknown and potentially toxic effects of supplements, this recommendation applies to foods as sources of nutrients—not to dietary supplements of individual nutrients.

☐ The consumption of salt-cured, salt-pickled, or smoked foods should be minimized.

☐ Alcoholic beverages should be consumed in moderation, if they are consumed at all.

Again, the centerpiece of these four guidelines, in terms of their practical daily application, is the importance of including whole grains, vegetables, and fruits in the diet, along with decreasing fat intake. Adoption of this dietary pattern results in increased consumption of fiber, vitamins A, C, and E, and other dietary components that may protect against the formation of cancer. Of particular note is the warning against relying on supplements to add dietary constituents that may help prevent cancer.

A comparison of the standard macrobiotic diet with these guidelines once again highlights the uncanny degree of agreement between the two. The emphases on whole grains and vegetables, and on decreasing fat intake can be seen as guiding principles for the prevention of cancer and other degenerative diseases.

These recommendations were repeated in March 1989 when the National Research Council (NRC), the working arm of the National Academy of Sciences, issued a subsequent report entitled *Diet and Health*. The 1989 report proposed broad changes in the modern diet in order to reduce the risk of heart disease and cancer. A special Committee on Diet and Health was established within the NRC to review the evidence linking diet with disease and to make dietary recommendations aimed at prevention. The Committee spent three years examining nearly 6,000 studies and issued a 1,400-page report that recommended increasing the intake of whole grains and other foods high in complex carbohydrates and fiber.

The Committee recommended that Americans approximately double their intake of these foods. The NRC also stated that reducing the amount of fat in the diet to below 30 percent of calories could lower the risk of heart disease by 20 percent. Increasing the intake of orange-yellow and leafy green vegetables high in beta-carotene could lower the risk of cancer of the colon, lung, and stomach.

AMERICAN CANCER SOCIETY DIETARY GUIDELINES

In 1984, the American Cancer Society (ACS) issued dietary guidelines for the first time in respect to the cause and prevention of cancer. Like the preceding recommendations, these guidelines point in the direction of the standard macrobiotic diet. In the ACS publication, *Nutrition and Cancer: Cause and Prevention,* we read:

> There is now good reason to suspect that dietary habits contribute to human cancer, but it is important to understand that the interpretation of both human population (epidemiologic) and laboratory data is very complex, and as yet does not allow clear-cut conclusions. . . . Foods may have constituents that cause or promote cancer on the one hand or protect against it on the other. No concrete dietary advice can be given that will guarantee prevention of any specific human cancer. The American Cancer Society nonetheless believes that there is sufficient inferential information to make a series of interim recommendations about nutrition that, in the judgment of experts, are likely to provide some measure of reducing cancer risk.

The ACS dietary recommendations, as presented in this publication, are:

- ☐ Avoid obesity.
- ☐ Cut down on total fat intake.
- ☐ Eat more high-fiber foods, such as whole grain cereals, fruits, and vegetables.
- ☐ Include foods rich in vitamins A and C in the daily diet.
- ☐ Include cruciferous vegetables, such as cabbage, broc-

coli, Brussels sprouts, kohlrabi, and cauliflower in the diet.

☐ Be moderate in consumption of alcoholic beverages.

☐ Be moderate in consumption of salt-cured, smoked, and nitrite-cured foods.

In the 1990 edition of *Cancer Facts and Figures*, published by the ACS, the section on cancer prevention lists diet as a key component of "primary prevention." Diet modification is one of the "steps that might be taken to avoid those factors that might lead to the development of cancer." The section on nutrition states:

> Risk for colon, breast, and uterine cancers increases in obese people. High-fat diets may contribute to the development of cancers of the breast, colon, and prostate. High-fiber foods may help reduce risk of colon cancer. A varied diet containing plenty of vegetables and fruits rich in vitamins A and C may reduce risk for a wide range of cancers. Salt-cured, smoked, and nitrite-cured foods have been linked to esophageal and stomach cancer. The heavy use of alcohol, especially when accompanied by cigarette smoking or chewing tobacco, increases risk of cancers of the mouth, larynx, throat, esophagus, and liver.

The report provides further information on the diet-cancer connection, stating that people who are 40 percent or more overweight have a higher risk of colon, breast, prostate, gall-bladder, ovarian, and uterine cancers, and that diets high in whole grains, vegetables, and other high-fiber foods (all of which are featured in the standard macrobiotic diet) may help reduce the risk of colon cancer. It also states that dark green and orange-yellow vegetables may help lower the risk of cancers of the lung, larynx, and esophagus.

The convergence of the standard macrobiotic diet and these preventive guidelines was pointed out in 1984 by the Congressional Subcommittee on Health and Long-Term Care. The Subcommittee investigated the dietary practices of several groups and concluded:

> The current macrobiotic diet is essentially an almost pure vegetarian diet as compared to the predominately

lacto-ovo-vegetarian diet primarily practiced by Seventh Day Adventists. The macrobiotic diet appears to be nutritionally adequate if the mix of foods proposed in the dietary recommendations are followed carefully. There is no apparent evidence of any nutritional deficiencies among current macrobiotic practices. . . . The diet would also be consistent with the recently released dietary guidelines of the National Academy of Sciences and the American Cancer Society in regard to possible reduction of cancer risks.

DIETARY GUIDELINES OF THE AMERICAN MEDICAL ASSOCIATION

The American Medical Association (AMA) also lent its general support to macrobiotics in the 1987 edition of the *American Medical Association Family Medical Guide*. In a section on special diets, the AMA reference guide states:

In the macrobiotic diet foods fall into two main groups, known as yin and yang (based on an Eastern principle of opposites), depending on where they have been grown, their texture, color, and composition. The general principle behind the macrobiotic diet is that foods biologically furthest away from us are better for us. Cereals therefore form the basis of the diet and fish is preferred to meat. Although fresh foods free of additives are preferred, no food is actually prohibited, in the belief that a craving for any food may reflect a genuine bodily need. In general, the macrobiotic diet is a healthful way of eating.

In its own revised dietary guidelines, the AMA recommended:

- ☐ Eat meat no more than once a day and choose fish or poultry over red meat.
- ☐ Bake or broil food rather than fry it and use polyunsaturated oils rather than butter, lard, or margarine.
- ☐ Cut down on salt, MSG, and other flavorings high in sodium.
- ☐ Eat more fiber including whole grain cereals, leafy green vegetables, and fruit.

"I'm Not Going to Die"

My story began on a beautiful September day in 1979, perfect for raking oak leaves. Feeling full of vim, vigor, and vitality, I had no reason to suspect I was anything but a specimen of health—not until my next–door neighbor told me about his prostate operation and the symptoms leading up to it. For days thereafter, I experienced his symptoms vicariously. When this happened, a voice within me said, "Go see the doctor and have a checkup." Invariably, my "better judgment" told me this was nonsense, forget it. After a month of debating with the "voice," I gave in, and made an appointment with my internist in Muskegon, Michigan, near where I live.

"What's the problem, Ed?" he inquired.

"Doctor, two years ago you told me my prostate was slightly enlarged and suggested you check it once a year. That's why I'm here."

While performing the examination, he remarked, "Ed, there's something hard there. I suggest you have a urologist check it." He didn't tell me he'd felt two tumors.

The urologist agreed there was "something hard there," didn't mention tumors, and recommended a biopsy. A week later I was shocked to learn I had prostate cancer. A bone scan followed. "Hot spots" showed up on my skull and pelvis. It was the doctor's opinion that the prostate cancer was in Stage II and the hot spots were either calcium deposits or arthritis. He recommended removal of the prostate—"and you'll be rid of the cancer." Scared as hell, I'd have agreed to anything.

At the suggestion of one of our sons, Dick, my wife, Jeanne, and I considered a second opinion and decided in favor of the Mayo Clinic. A group of three doctors reviewed my medical record; next, my prostate was examined. Then came blood and urine tests and, finally, a bone scan. My last stop was the office of the urologist in charge of my case. He'd already received the reports on the tests and scan. After studying the reports, he looked up at me and said, "Ed, no operation for you."

That wasn't what I'd expected to hear, and I remained speechless for a moment. "No? Why not?"

"Ed, unless we do a bone biopsy, we don't know for certain it's malignant. However, we feel the odds lean heavily in that direction. If we operate, and it is cancer, the cancer will metastasize much faster. We don't know how to cure it, but we can slow it down either of two ways: castrate you or prescribe female hormone pills. I 'guesstimate' this would give you another ten years." Of course, I took the hormone pills.

During the next two years, the cancer remained dormant in my prostate, skull, and pelvis, but then metastasized to my spine, some ribs, and left thighbone.

One evening my eldest son, David, came to visit me. "Dad, you probably wonder why I've come to visit you on a week night. I'll be frank; I'm terribly upset these days because I harbor the thought you're dying. I don't want to lose you. Not now. I'm just getting to know you." He hugged me; tears flowed down his face onto my cheek. Then I cried, too.

After wiping my eyes, I said, "David, I'm not going to die for a long time yet."

Wiping the tears from his eyes, he said, "Don't you think so, Dad?"

The truth is, until that very moment I was resigned to the fact I was dying. Those words, "We don't know how to cure it," had me convinced. Then a strange thing happened. I suddenly became obsessed with a strong desire to live. From then on I prayed daily for the strength, the ways, and the means to overcome the cancer.

At Bible study class one Saturday morning a friend gave me an article from the *Saturday Evening Post* about a doctor who had recovered from prostate and bone cancer by adhering to a diet of whole grains, vegetables, sea vegetables, seeds, and nuts. It was called macrobiotics. It seemed too incredible to be given credence.

Nevertheless, I couldn't put it out of my mind. Over and over, I asked myself, what's there to lose by trying it? Finally, with Jeanne's encouragement, I decided to go for it.

At the Kushi Foundation in Brookline, Massachusetts, Edward Esko, a senior teacher, discussed with me a diet typical of that which had helped the recovered doctor. He also stressed the importance of daily exercise. Before leaving, Jeanne and I took cooking lessons.

During the next twelve months, I adhered strictly to the diet. My only supplements were daily exercise and prayers (others' and my own).

Jeanne had become my faithful "watchdog." If I so much as looked at a cut of red meat or poultry in a butcher's showcase, a picture of a martini (dry), or that joint with the Big Arch, she stared me down and gave me a sermon on the spot. We both shared in the cooking and accumulated a library full of cookbooks.

At mass, we often sing, "Great Things Happen When God Mixes With Us." How true it is—September 12, 1983, three years after discovering I had cancer, one year to the day on the macrobiotic diet, doctors at the University of Chicago gave me a clean bill of health: a bone scan, prostate biopsy, blood and urine tests disclosed no signs of cancer cells.

Source: Ed Hanley, "The Hand on My Shoulder," *One Peaceful World*, Spring, 1990.

☐ Eat no more than four eggs a week.
☐ For dessert or a snack choose fresh fruit rather than cookies, cakes, or puddings.

THE CHINA STUDY

New evidence from an ongoing study of diet and health in China is challenging many nutritional concepts and offering further scientific support for the health-enhancing potential of the standard macrobiotic diet. It also suggests that preventive guidelines like the preceding may be too modest, and that more substantial dietary changes may be necessary to reduce the risk of cancer and other degenerative illnesses. The study was started in 1983 by T. Colin Campbell, a nutritional biochemist at Cornell University, and is based on data collected from 6,500 people in China. Preliminary findings from the study, which is the largest epidemiological survey of its kind so far, were published in June 1990 by Cornell University Press and include the following discoveries:

☐ *To lower the risk of cancer and heart disease, dietary fat may need to be reduced to far below the 30 percent of calories recommended by the National Academy of Sciences and other leading public health agencies.* Data from the study suggest that it may be necessary to lower fat intake to 10 to 15 percent of calories—more in the range of the standard macrobiotic diet—in order to substantially reduce the risk of these illnesses.

☐ *Overconsumption of animal protein could play a role in*

the development of cancer, heart disease, and diabetes. Among the people who were surveyed, those who consumed the most animal protein were found to have the highest rates of these diseases. In general, Americans eat about 30 percent more protein than the Chinese, with about 70 percent of it coming from animal sources. (People in China consume an average of 7 percent of their protein from animal sources.) This finding suggests that the macrobiotic emphasis on eating vegetable rather than animal protein could lower the risk of cancer, heart disease, and diabetes.

☐ *The risk of breast and female reproductive cancers may be increased by eating a diet high in calories, protein, fat, and calcium during childhood.* This dietary pattern, which is typical of the modern American diet, promotes rapid growth in childhood and could be a major factor in causing menstruation to start at an earlier age. Women who were surveyed were found to begin menstruating three to six years later than American women and to have much lower rates of these types of cancer.

☐ *Dairy products are not necessary to prevent osteoporosis.* As we will see in the discussion of calcium presented later, studies have shown that countries where little or no dairy food is consumed have lower rates of osteoporosis than do countries where large amounts of dairy food are eaten. A similar finding emerged from the China study. Dairy foods are normally not a part of the Chinese diet, and osteoporosis was rare among the people who were surveyed. As with people who consume a standard macrobiotic diet, the people in the survey derive most of their calcium from vegetable sources.

The data also suggest that a high cholesterol level may predispose one to cancer, heart disease, and diabetes. As Dr. Campbell stated in an interview, "So far, we've seen that plasma cholesterol is a good predictor of the kinds of diseases people are going to get. Those with higher cholesterol levels are prone to the diseases of affluence — cancer, heart disease, and diabetes." Cholesterol levels in China were found to range from 88 to 165 milligrams per 100 milliliters of blood, similar to the range among people eating a standard macrobiotic diet, and much lower than average in the United Sates. The researchers also found that the rates of colon cancer were lowest among people who had the lowest cholesterol levels. These results suggest that high consumption of dairy products and other animal foods has a major influence on higher cholesterol levels and a higher incidence of the aforementioned diseases.

Evidence from the study also suggests that meat and other animal foods are not necessary to prevent anemia. The main sources of iron in the Chinese diet are vegetable foods, and the researchers found little evidence of iron-deficiency anemia among those surveyed. There was no evidence from the study that fiber interfered with the absorption of iron; in fact, persons who ate the most fiber were found to have the highest levels of iron in the blood.

Dr. Campbell summarized the preliminary results of the study in an interview: "We are basically a vegetarian species and should be eating a wide variety of plant foods and minimizing our intake of animal foods." The preliminary results of this ongoing diet and health study seem to indicate that a diet along the lines of the standard macrobiotic diet can be of substantial benefit in reducing the incidence of the major degenerative diseases of our time.

A NUTRITIONAL OVERVIEW OF THE MACROBIOTIC DIET

In order to determine whether the macrobiotic diet is nutritionally adequate and can promote health and well-being, it is necessary to understand this diet, not only as it is described in books, but, more importantly, as it is practiced. The standard macrobiotic diet approximates usual macrobiotic eating patterns and is based upon principles fundamental to the macrobiotic way of life. Therefore, the diet can serve as a reference with which to evaluate nutritional adequacy.

It is important to realize that while the standard macrobiotic diet is often described in fixed terms, it encompasses a wide range of eating patterns, varying in order to create balance with one's environment and physical and mental conditions. Thus, it is no more rigid than any other set of guidelines or standards describing an ideal or norm; in fact, since it embodies the principles of change and balance, it is perhaps less rigid than many.

The general guidelines, according to which the standard macrobiotic diet has been designed, are used as a framework within which each individual can approach the macrobiotic way of eating. As a basic plan for human nutrition, these dietary guidelines are no more arbitrary or inflexible than are the "four basic food groups." The guidelines follow:

- [ ] Each meal should consist primarily of vegetable-quality food.
- [ ] The principal foods around which meals are designed should be whole cereal grains, supplemented with legumes (beans).
- [ ] Vegetables should be selected in harmony with the seasons and the environment, and, in general, should be cooked.
- [ ] Sea vegetables are another important food that should be eaten on a daily basis.
- [ ] Fruit and nuts should also be chosen with seasonal and environmental considerations. Give preference to those that are in season and are indigenous to a climate similar to the one in which you live.
- [ ] Vegetable-quality oils and unrefined sea salt should be among the primary seasonings.
- [ ] Beverages, seasonings, and condiments should be used only if grown in a climate similar to the one in which you live.

To summarize the underlying principles, the emphasis on whole cereal grains underscores the importance of consuming foods that are as unrefined and unprocessed as possible. Also emphasized is the central role of vegetable-quality over animal-quality foods.

When determining the nutritional adequacy of a diet, the standards most often used in the United States are the Recommended Dietary Allowances (RDA), published by the National Academy of Sciences. International standards are based on the recommendations put forth by the Food and Agricultural Organization and the World Health Organization (FAO/WHO). Both of these standards will be referred to when describing the standard macrobiotic diet and its nutritional adequacy.

We are using the RDA and the FAO/WHO standards as reference intakes even though they have purposely been set high. The National Academy of Science's explanation that the "RDA should not be confused with requirements" and, "RDA are estimated to exceed the requirements of most individuals, and thereby ensure that the needs of nearly all are met" applies equally well to the FAO/WHO standards for most of the world's population.

In addressing the question of the nutritional adequacy of the standard macrobiotic diet, we deal with two questions:

1. How much of a given nutrient is required?
2. Does the standard macrobiotic diet provide at least that amount?

Protein

It is a common misconception that predominantly vegetarian diets are protein deficient. This view arises from the belief that animal foods are synonymous with protein in the diet. In the "four food groups," the "protein group" emphasizes meat, poultry, and fish, and only begrudgingly acknowledges peanut butter and beans as sources. While this idea is common, it is not necessarily correct. Indeed, the perception that vegetarian diets are deficient in protein ignores the fact that Americans often consume amounts of protein that are more than twice the RDA.

The RDA states that the allowance for protein intake is approximately 0.8 grams of protein per kilogram of body weight per day. For an average (65 kilogram) male, this means 53 grams per day, and for an average (55 kilogram) female, this would be 44 grams. The RDA provides two safety measures: one to adjust for the variations in protein quality (relative amounts of the various essential amino acids), and the usual increase to cover the range of requirements encountered among different individuals. Thus, in terms of the RDA, protein quality and completeness — the presence of all the essential amino acids — are generally root issues for most diets.

The FAO/WHO has established figures comparable to the RDAs for daily recommended intakes of protein — 37 grams for an adult man, and 39 grams for an adult woman. In addition, the FAO/WHO provides an alternative standard, which is that diets should contain at least 7 percent of calories as protein. It is interesting to note the difference between the RDA and the FAO/WHO standards, and wonder about the possible reasons why they differ. Regardless, however, of which standard is used, the standard macrobiotic diet is protein-sufficient. It is a truism that virtually all diets of "mixed foods," whether vegetarian or not, will provide 10 to 14 percent of calories as protein, exceeding the standard put forth by FAO/WHO. The protein content of typical foods is listed in Table 4.1.

The absolute amount of protein eaten by persons consuming a standard macrobiotic diet depends, of course, upon the amount of food eaten. An analysis of the protein intake recorded by persons eating a normal macrobiotic diet of three meals per day demonstrated that this was, indeed, the case, and that protein deficiency was not a problem. Even with a relatively limited intake of around 1,600 calories per day, the amount of protein eaten will approximate or exceed both the RDAs and the FAO/WHO standards.

Vitamin C (Ascorbic Acid)

Generally speaking, fruits and leafy green vegetables provide most of the vitamin C in any diet. Broccoli, cauliflower, and watercress are some of the many vitamin-C-rich foods commonly included in the standard macrobiotic diet. In fact, only a relatively small portion—half a cup of kale or lightly cooked turnip greens, for example—approaches or exceeds the FAO/WHO standards (30 milligrams per day) and the RDA (60 milligrams) for vitamin C. Clearly, the standard macrobiotic diet, which includes many other sources of vitamin C, is not deficient in this nutrient. On the contrary, the calculated intakes of vitamin C recorded by those who eat a macrobiotic diet generally exceed the recommended allowances by 50 to 100 percent.

Riboflavin (Vitamin B_2)

Almost 40 percent of the riboflavin in most American diets comes from dairy food—rarely consumed on a macrobiotic

Table 4.1   **Protein Content of Various Foods**

	Food	Protein Content*
Whole Cereal Grains	Brown rice, various types	7.4–7.5
	Wheat, various	9.4–14.0
	Oats	13.0
	Barley, various	8.2–8.9
	Rye, various	12.1–12.7
	Millet, various	9.9–12.7
	Buckwheat, various	11.0–14.5
	Corn, various	8.2–8.9
	Sorghum	11.0–12.7
Beans and Bean Products	Azuki beans	21.5
	Broad beans, various	25.1–26.0
	Kidney beans	20.2
	Lima beans	20.4
	Mung beans	23.0–24.2
	Peas, dried, various	21.7–24.1
	Soybeans, various	34.1–34.3
	Natto	16.9
	Tempeh, various	18.3–48.7
	Tofu	7.8
Seeds and Nuts	Various	11.0–29.7
Meat and Poultry	Beef, various	13.6–21.8
	Pork, various	9.1–21.5
	Chicken, various	14.5–23.4
	Other birds and poultry	18.5–25.3
	Eggs, various	12.9–13.9
Dairy Food	Cheese, various	13.6–27.5
Fish and Seafood	Fishes, various	16.4–25.4
	Shellfish, various	10.6–24.8
	Seafood, various	15.0–20.0

*Grams per 3.5-ounce typical serving.
Sources: U.S. Department of Agriculture and Japan Nutritionist Association.

diet. However, leafy green vegetables such as kale and mustard greens contain as much riboflavin per average serving as dairy food. Whole grains and beans are also good sources of riboflavin.

Adequacy of riboflavin intake is determined in terms of total caloric intake, since the standard is given as 0.57 milligrams per 1,000 calories. Riboflavin is so ubiquitous in foods that frank riboflavin deficiency has not easily been detected in free-living populations. Indeed, it is unclear what the consequences of consuming inadequate riboflavin might be. In any case, riboflavin intake on a standard macrobiotic diet easily meets the RDA and FAO/WHO standards.

Vitamin B_{12}

Protein and vitamin B_{12} are the nutrients most often perceived as being deficient in any predominantly vegetarian diet. This opinion ignores some basic facts about vitamin B_{12}. It is commonly taught and believed that animal food products are the only dietary sources of vitamin B_{12}, a required nutrient for virtually all animals. There are, however, many species of animals that live entirely on vegetable-quality food. How is it that such vegetarian animal species have enough vitamin B_{12} for their physiological needs?

Cows, for instance, eat only vegetable-quality food, provide a major portion of typical American diets, and are considered to be good sources of vitamin B_{12} for humans. What is the source of the cows' vitamin B_{12}?

The missing link is fundamental to the understanding of what constitutes a good dietary source of vitamin B_{12}. In fact, virtually all the available vitamin B_{12} is originally synthesized by microorganisms such as bacteria or mold. Cows get their vitamin B_{12} from bacteria that reside in their gastrointestinal tract. Interestingly, other animals (including humans) may have substantial portions of their vitamin B_{12} requirement met through contamination of their food by bacteria, as when dirty food is eaten. While the gastrointestinal bacteria in humans supply only negligible amounts of vitamin B_{12}, foods that contain B_{12}-producing microorganisms provide adequate amounts of that vitamin.

The standard macrobiotic diet includes several foods in this category. Some of these foods have microorganisms attached to them as a result of fermentation. Primary examples of fermented foods in the macrobiotic diet are the soybean products miso, natto, and tempeh, traditional foods in the Far East. Because of the extremely small requirements for vitamin

B_{12} (the RDA and FAO/WHO standards for adults are 3 and 2 micrograms, respectively), these foods are adequate sources.

In addition to these vegetable-quality sources of vitamin B_{12}, the standard macrobiotic diet does permit the eating of animal foods. Consumption of fish from time to time more than adequately meets daily needs for vitamin B_{12} because this vitamin may be stored in the liver.

Vitamin A (Retinol and Beta-Carotene)

Because of the lack of vitamin A in brown rice, some nutritionists believe that a macrobiotic diet is lacking in this vitamin. The standard macrobiotic diet easily meets recommended intake for this nutrient, the consumption of which has been identified as an aid in the prevention and treatment of cancer. People who eat macrobiotically regularly consume vegetables with a high beta-carotene content. These include leafy green vegetables, as well as yellowish-orange vegetables such as carrots or winter squash. Beta-carotene intake on a macrobiotic diet is probably greater than that on a typical American diet.

The RDA for vitamin A is 1,000 micrograms of retinol, 6,000 micrograms of beta-carotene, or some combination of the two. Similarly, the FAO/WHO standard is 750 micrograms of retinol or its equivalent in beta-carotene. This amount is contained in one small carrot, or in two-thirds of a cup of cooked kale.

Vitamin D

Eating fish on a regular basis can help provide vitamin D in the macrobiotic diet. The only group for which vitamin D deficiency might be a problem is rapidly growing children. For adolescents and adults, more than enough vitamin D for metabolic needs is synthesized within the body through the action of ultraviolet rays shining on the skin.

There have been scattered cases in which children whose parents considered themselves to be eating macrobiotically, developed overt signs of vitamin D deficiency. Such problems do not occur when one keeps in mind the important macrobiotic principle of eating a wide variety of foods. These parents seem to have neglected to include plenty of fresh vegetables; furthermore, there was an overuse of salt and salty condiments. To correct a severe vitamin D deficiency, it would be necessary to complement the diet of the growing child with a good source of this nutrient, such as cod or other fish liver oils, until the proper dietary patterns are established.

A number of such cases also occurred following long periods of minimal exposure to the sun, a condition easily enough remedied by taking children outside on a regular basis.

In no case where the macrobiotic diet has been flexible and accurately applied has there been a report of rickets, a condition caused by a lack of vitamin D.

Calcium

One reason for the idea that calcium intake may be a problem on the macrobiotic diet is the notion that dietary calcium must come from dairy foods. This misconception is largely a cultural phenomenon, unique to the United States and a few other industrialized countries. With few exceptions throughout the rest of the world, dairy food is rarely consumed in the quantities thought necessary by most Americans. Oddly, osteoporosis, the disease often regarded as being due primarily to calcium deficiency, is relatively common in industrialized nations, and occurs less frequently in the Third World, where dairy foods are not widely consumed.

The standard macrobiotic diet, in fact, includes several good sources of calcium such as sea vegetables, leafy green vegetables, beans and nuts. Tofu is another good source of calcium. The calcium content of various foods is shown in Table 4.2. Average calcium intake on the macrobiotic diet is in the range considered adequate by the FAO/WHO (400 to 500 milligrams per day).

Because whole grains and vegetables make up a major portion of the standard macrobiotic diet, concern has been expressed about the binding of calcium by phytase or oxalates contained in some of these foods. (It appears that refining of food removes these compounds, apparently making more calcium available for use by the body.) Although this inhibition

Bed to Wheelchair to Cane to Health

In April 1980, I had a diagnostic procedure done to determine the cause of the excessive and prolonged menstrual bleeding I was experiencing. The doctor discovered a malignant tumor—a carcinosarcoma in the connective tissue on the wall of the uterus. I was given twenty radiation treatments, a radium implant, hormone medication, and both oral and intravenous chemotherapy. In August 1980, the doctor performed a radical hysterectomy and a "bilateral salpingo oophorectomy."—the removal of my ovaries. I continued to take chemotherapy.

In May 1982, I started having pain in the lower back, and despite medication, it got progressively worse. I could neither sit nor lie down. In August, after a few days of standing up day and night, sleeping only on my husband's shoulder in a standing position, I went to an orthopedist. He confirmed a compression fracture and noted also that my vertebrae were partially collapsed. In order to prevent a total collapse of the vertebrae, I was put into a brace that extended from above the chest to the pelvic area around the back.

The pain got worse and spread to my legs. I could no longer stand. My husband put me in a reclining chair and gave me strong pain-killers around the clock. Nothing stopped the pain.

In September I was carried to the hospital for more x-rays and scans. In addition to the compression fracture and the partially collapsed vertebrae, these pictures showed cancer on the lumbar spine, cancer on the thoracic spine, and multiple metastatic deposits on both lungs.

I was given radiation again (a series of five treatments), then chemotherapy, then five more radiation treatments, then more chemotherapy. The usual program was ten rounds of chemotherapy, given at three- to four-week intervals. I was tired, weak, nauseated, and in pain.

In January 1983, after four cycles of chemotherapy, x-rays and scans were taken again. The tests showed that there was increased activity and progression of the cancer in the spine, and unchanged metastatic cancer in both lungs.

Towards the end of January, while opening the mail, I cut my finger on an envelope. Because my blood levels were so depressed from the chemotherapy, I was unable to fight the infection that set in. The paper-cut resulted in a ten-day hospital stay, including four blood transfusions, massive doses of intravenous antibiotics, and three days in isolation. It was decided that the chemotherapy I was getting was too strong; I would be put on something less toxic.

It was then that I knew that conventional medicine was not going to work for me. I did some research on alternative methods, and I chose macrobiotics. Dr. Sattilaro's book *Recalled By Life* was a great inspiration to me. I felt that if he could get well on such a program, I could too. In mid-February I started to wean myself away from meat, dairy products, fruit, and sugar, and to reduce to zero the thirty-eight pills I was taking daily. By the end of February, I was on the macrobiotic diet.

I began the diet in a hospital bed, a wheelchair, and a brace. In a short while, I started walking with a walker, then with a cane. In April, a urinary problem that had plagued me for three years (a result of the original radiation) disappeared. In mid-May I took off the brace. On May 22, I walked up and down my block all by myself.

In June, I put away my wig; my hair, which had all fallen out from the chemotherapy, had grown back enough to be presentable. I returned the hospital bed. I started driving again. I resumed my studies towards my master's degree. In six months, I changed from a sick, depressed, pill-popping invalid to a happy, optimistic, and very grateful pain-free person.

The side effects of the diet have been mostly positive. I have had a few bouts with diarrhea, fatigue, flaky skin, and other non-debilitating forms of "discharge." On the positive side, I enjoy good health, good energy, and perfect bodily functions, such as appetite, sleep, elimination, and mental acuity. And I really enjoy the food—my whole family does, too.

Although I take no treatments or medications, I continue to see my oncologist periodically for check-ups. She says that I am doing very well.

I have now been practicing macrobiotics for eight years. I have completed a Master of Science degree in nutrition. I am doing nutritional consulting and helping many people with all kinds of degenerative diseases and other illnesses to improve their health. In addition, I teach macrobiotic cooking classes and lecture throughout the New York-New Jersey area.

I attribute the reversal of my cancer solely to macrobiotics, and I hope that my story will be a source of hope and inspiration to others.

Source: Elaine Nussbaum, "From Pill-Popping to Pain-Free," *East West Journal*, May, 1984, and *Recovery: From Cancer to Health through Macrobiotics*, Japan Publications, 1986.

Table 4.2   **Calcium Content of Various Foods**

	Food	Calcium Content*
Leafy Green Vegetables	Beet greens	100
	Collard greens	203
	Daikon greens	190
	Kale	179
	Mustard greens	183
	Parsley	200
	Spinach	98
	Watercress	90
Beans and Bean Products	Broad beans	100
	Chick-peas	150
	Kidney beans	130
	Soybeans	226
	Miso	140
	Natto	103
	Tofu	128
Grains	Buckwheat	114
Sea Vegetables†	Agar-agar	400
	Arame	1,170
	Dulse	567
	Hijiki	1,400
	Kombu	800
	Nori	400
	Wakame	1,300
Seeds and Nuts†	Sesame seeds	1,160
	Sunflower seeds	140
	Sweet almonds	282
	Brazil nuts	186
	Hazelnuts	209
Fish and Seafood	Carp	50
	Haddock	23
	Salmon	79
	Shortneck clams	80
	Oyster	94
Dairy Food	Cow's milk	118
	Eggs	65
	Goat's milk	120
	Cheese, various	250-850
	Yogurt	120

*Milligrams per 3.5-ounce typical serving.
†A typical serving will usually be from about one-fourth to one-half this amount.
Sources: U.S. Department of Agriculture and Japan Nutritionist Association.

of calcium absorption by phytase has been demonstrated experimentally, it is the general view of nutritionists that "the importance of phytic acid (phytase) as an anti-calcifying factor in human nutrition has not been established."

Iron

Adequate stores of iron are needed for the formation of red blood cells. Because animal food is commonly perceived to be the best source of dietary iron, the macrobiotic diet has been criticized for potentially leading to the development of iron-deficiency anemia. In fact, about as much dietary iron in the American diet is provided by grain, fruit, or vegetables as by meat.

The American diet is low in iron compared to diets worldwide, and anemia may, indeed, be the most widespread nutritional deficiency disease in the United States. The American diet is relatively deficient in iron because of the highly refined nature of the diet. The iron content of various foods is shown in Table 4.3.

One of the principles of the standard macrobiotic diet is the consumption of foods in as whole and unrefined a state as possible. Since refining of grain removes much of its iron, any one food in the macrobiotic diet, compared to its counterpart in the U.S. diet, probably contains as much or more iron. Also, most of the sea vegetables included in the macrobiotic diet are particularly rich sources of iron.

It is evident that for most people on a macrobiotic diet, iron intake is not a problem. Possible exceptions to this are pregnant and lactating women who have an increased iron need because of the growing fetus or newborn. In these cases, to ensure adequate iron intake, the standard macrobiotic diet is adjusted to include a larger proportion of sea vegetables and other iron-rich foods, and emphasis is placed on the use of cast-iron cookware.

PREVENTIVE NUTRITION

The standard macrobiotic diet, when examined for its nutritional adequacy, is clearly an acceptable diet by any stan-

Table 4.3   Iron Content of Various Foods

	Food	Iron Content*
Whole Grains	Buckwheat	3.1
	Millet	6.8
	Oats	4.6
	Soba	5.0
	Whole wheat, various	3.1-3.3
Beans	Azuki beans	4.8
	Chickpeas	6.9
	Lentils	6.8
	Soybeans	7.0
Green Leafy Vegetables	Beet greens	3.3
	Dandelion greens	3.1
	Mustard greens	3.0
	Parsley	6.2
	Spinach	3.1
	Swiss chard	3.2
Seeds†	Pumpkin seeds	11.2
	Sesame seeds	10.5
	Sunflower seeds	7.1
Sea Vegetables†	Arame	12.0
	Dulse	6.3
	Hijiki	29.0
	Kombu	15.0
	Nori	23.0
	Wakame	13.0
Fish and Seafood	Herring	1.1
	Sardines	2.9
	Abalone	2.4
	Oyster	5.5
Meat and Poultry	Beef	3.6
	Chicken	1.6
	Egg yolk	6.3
	Beef liver	6.5
	Calf liver	8.7
	Chicken liver, various	7.9
Refined Sugar	Molasses	6.0

*Milligrams per 3.5-ounce typical serving.

†A typical serving will usually be from one-fourth to one-half this amount.

Sources: U.S. Department of Agriculture and Japan Nutritionist Association.

dard. As long as the principles of macrobiotics are applied in choosing one's diet, nutritional deficiencies will not be a problem. In fact, if "good nutrition" means not only avoiding deficiency diseases, but also promoting good health, malnutrition ("bad nutrition") probably occurs much less frequently in people who eat a standard macrobiotic diet than in those who eat a typical American diet.

The macrobiotic diet is an optimal example of a diet that can prevent degenerative disease. This potential has not only been supported by the United States Dietary Goals, the National Academy of Sciences Report on Cancer, and the other preventive guidelines mentioned before, but it has also been demonstrated.

In surveys conducted among people who follow a macrobiotic diet, medical researchers have examined the role of diet in altering the physiological risk factors for cardiovascular disease. Two risk factors have been studied: blood pressure and blood cholesterol levels. These are considered risk factors for heart disease. (The higher the levels, the greater the probability of developing heart disease.)

It has been unequivocally demonstrated that blood cholesterol levels of people on a macrobiotic diet (averaging 126 milligrams of cholesterol per deciliter of blood) are much lower than those of people consuming an American diet (averaging more than 200 milligrams per deciliter), even after taking into account other factors that influence cholesterol levels. Similarly, people on a macrobiotic diet have much lower blood pressures (averaging 106/60) than would be expected in the general United States population. Since these trends appear to continue throughout life, it is highly probable that very few people who eat a macrobiotic diet will develop heart disease.

A recent study has shown that diet and lifestyle can reverse arterial blockages that are the chief causes of heart attacks and strokes. The study, known as "The Lifestyle Heart Trial," was conducted by cardiologist Dean Ornish and his colleagues at the University of California at San Francisco and published in *The Lancet* in July 1990. The researchers found that volunteers who ate a very low-fat, primarily vegetarian diet that excluded poultry, high-fat dairy products, red meat, oils, and fats were able to partially clear their blocked arteries. "Comprehensive lifestyle changes may be able to bring about regression of even severe coronary arteriosclerosis after only one year," the study reported. Claude L'enfant, director of the National Heart, Lung, and Blood Institute, said the most interesting aspect of the study was the finding that changes in diet alone "can be just as effective in reversing blocked arteries as cholesterol-lowering drugs." However, the researchers cautioned that "adherence to this lifestyle program needs to be very good for overall regression to occur, although more moderate changes have some beneficial effect."

Awareness of the relationship between diet and heart disease has progressed from initial suspicion that the modern high-fat diet is a primary causative factor, to the recognition that a low-fat, high-fiber diet, similar to the standard macrobiotic diet, would help prevent heart disease. Most recently it has been discovered that a more naturally balanced diet can actually reverse certain forms of heart disease. The Lifestyle Heart Trial adds substantial weight to the macrobiotic idea that the types of foods that prevent a particular disease are also those that help in recovering from it. Prevention and recovery are not separate issues. A similar evolution is occurring in the awareness of the relationship between diet and cancer.

As we have seen, public awareness of this relationship is largely at the second stage of this process: the recognition that the modern diet promotes cancer and that a naturally balanced diet along the lines of macrobiotics can help prevent it. In the near future, as the cancer-inhibiting properties of foods such as whole grains, beans, orange-yellow and cruciferous vegetables, and sea vegetables are better understood, recognition that the macrobiotic diet can help not only in the prevention of cancer, but also in the recovery from it, will become commonplace. Public health policy can then evolve beyond the realm of prevention and into the dimension of recommending a prudent diet along the lines of macrobiotics for persons who develop cancer.

5

A Unifying Principle

In order to solve the problem of cancer, and create a cancer-free world in the future, we need a holistic model that explains—in common terms—the origin and cause of the disease. Although epidemiological studies are beginning to hint at the dietary causes of cancer, our modern understanding of health and sickness is not, for the most part, based on a comprehensive view of man and the universe. The modern view lacks a unifying principle that explains how human beings interact with their environment and how daily food serves as the intermediary between the two.

When our view is fragmentary and partial—rather than holistic and unifying—the impact of diet, in terms of its practical application, can easily be diluted. For example, certain compounds in foods that prevent cancer—beta carotene, for instance—have been identified and subsequently produced in capsule form. By concentrating on the anti-cancer effects of specific compounds, we sometimes miss the overwhelming significance of the dietary pattern as a whole in promoting or inhibiting cancer. As a result, our recommendations for preventing cancer may not be as comprehensive or effective as they could be.

The principle of yin and yang—which underlies the practice of macrobiotics—provides a unified view of human life and health, as well as a theoretical framework for understanding the origin and cause of cancer and other illnesses. Let us see how this principle applies to the problem of cancer, starting with an explanation of the principle itself.

THEORETICAL FRAMEWORK

If we observe the things around us, we see that they are made up of numerous complementary and opposite aspects. A chair, for example, is composed of legs that project downward and a seat and back that extend in the opposite direction. Each section of the chair—as well as the chair as a whole—contains an upper and lower part, a left and right side, a top and bottom, and an inside and outside.

Similar relationships exist in a book. It is composed of an outside cover and an inside text. It also has a front and back cover; usually the front cover is more bold and simple, while the back is more understated and detailed. When we open a book, it divides into left- and right-hand pages, and each page has a front and a back side. A book itself is defined by complementary opposites: for example, by its left and right and upper and lower borders, and by its first and last pages. On each page, there are many complementary relationships, such as those between text and illustrations, printed type and blank space, headings and text, words and punctuation, and many others. A book also has a duration, or lifespan, that is defined by its beginning and end.

Books, like everything else, do not exist in isolation. They exist in relation to other things in the environment. These relationships are also defined by complementary opposites. If we compare books, for example, we see that some are thick, others thin; some are large, others small; some reach a large audience, while others do not; and some have a lasting impact while the influence of others is relatively short-lived.

The biological world is also governed by similar relationships. There are complementary distinctions between plant and animal life, between more biologically developed species and less developed species, and between species that live in water and those that live on land. In the human body, the two branches of the autonomic nervous system—the sympathetic and the parasympathetic—work in an antagonistic yet complementary manner to control the body's automatic functions. The endocrine system operates in a similar manner. The pancreas, as we saw earlier, secretes insulin, which lowers the blood sugar level, and also secretes anti-insulin, which causes it to rise. The movements of the heart and lungs, digestive, endocrine, and other organs and glands continuously alternate between expansion and contraction. The rhythms of daily life—waking and sleeping, appetite and fullness, and movement and rest—also represent the alternation of opposites.

Actually, everything in the universe has a similar nature. All things appear and disappear, ebb and flow, and move back and forth between opposite conditions. Reality is a unified field of countless interrelationships, all of which are defined and governed by complementary opposites.

YIN AND YANG

If we make a list of all of the complementary opposites that we can identify in ourselves and the world around us, we will start to notice certain similarities. Let us take the distinction between expansion and contraction and large and small as an example. In terms of position, expansive force tends to push things toward the outside or periphery, while contracting force causes them to gather at the center. A peripheral position is, therefore, a function of expansion, while a central position is created by contraction. Expansive force also causes atoms and molecules to separate, and thus produces less density and a lighter weight. Contraction bunches atoms and molecules together and creates greater density and weight. Largeness is, therefore, a product of expansion and smallness, of contraction.

We can also analyze directions of movement from the perspective of yin and yang. Movement in an upward direction means movement away from the center of the earth, while downward movement implies movement toward the center. Thus, upward movement can be linked with the qualities of expansion, and downward movement with contraction. Centrifugal force, which is defined as movement away from a center of rotation, is also a more expansive quality, while centrip-

etal force, which is defined as movement toward a center of
rotation, is more contractive.

In Table 5.1, a variety of attributes are classified into yin
and yang. We can see that all complementary opposites can
be grouped into two categories. Physical attributes—temperature, size, weight, physical structure, color, wavelength, etc.—
yield numerous complementary tendencies that display either
a stronger tendency toward more expansive, centrifugal force,
or toward more contractive, centripetal force. Thousands of

Table 5.1   Examples of Yin and Yang

Characteristic	Yin($\triangledown$)	Yang($\triangle$)
Atomic particle	electron	proton
Attitude	more gentle, passive	more aggressive, active
Biological	more vegetable quality	more animal quality
Climate	temperate, colder	tropical, warmer
Direction	ascent, vertical, outward	descent, horizontal, inward
Flavor	sweet	salty
Food preparation	less cooked	more cooked
Form	longer, thinner	shorter, thicker
Function	diffusion	fusion
Humidity	more wet	more dry
Light	darker	brighter
Movement	more inactive, slower	more active, faster
Nerves	peripheral, orthosympathetic	central, para- sympathetic
Organ structure	more hollow, expansive	more dense, compacted
Position	more outward, peripheral	more inward, central
Sex	female	male
Shape	more expansive	more contracted
Size	larger	smaller
Temperature	colder	hotter
Tendency	expansion	contraction
Texture	softer	harder
Vibration	shorter wave, higher frequency	longer wave, lower frequency
Weight	lighter	heavier
Work	more psychological, mental	more physical, social

years ago, these complementary forces were seen as the most basic manifestations of the universe itself, and were given the names "yin" and "yang." Although these terms were first used in China, the concept they represent is not particularly Oriental. A similar understanding can be found in ancient cultures throughout the world.

ORIGIN AND CAUSE OF DISEASE

Some sicknesses are caused by an overly expanding tendency; others result from an overly contracting tendency; some sicknesses result from the combination of both extremes.

An example of a more yang sickness is a headache caused when the tissues and cells of the brain contract and press against each other, resulting in pressure and pain; a more yin headache arises when the tissues and cells press against each other as a result of being overexpanded and swollen. A stroke caused by constriction of the arteries that supply the brain is an example of a more yang sickness; while a stroke caused by hemorrhaging is a more yin disorder.

Cancer is characterized by a rapid increase in cells, and, in this respect, is a more expansive or yin phenomenon. However, the cause of cancer is more complex. Cancer can appear almost anywhere in the body: at the periphery of the body on the skin, or deep inside in the brain, liver, uterus, or bones. It can also develop in the upper body, in the breasts, for example, or in the lower body, such as in the cervix or prostate. Each type of cancer has a slightly different cause.

The distinction between prostate and breast cancer offers an example of the way that yin and yang influence the disease. Recently, female hormones have been used to temporarily inhibit prostate cancer. At the same time, male hormones have been found to have a controlling effect with certain types of breast cancer. Suppose, however, that female hormones were given to women with estrogen-dependent tumors. That would cause their cancers to develop more rapidly, and that is why estrogen-based contraceptives are associated with a higher risk of certain types of breast cancer. Similarly, the male hormone testosterone accelerates the growth of prostate cancer, and that is why doctors sometimes recommend orchidectomy, the surgical removal of the testicles, to slow the growth of the disease.

The influence of yin and yang can also be seen deep within each cell at the level of genes and chromosomes. More yin genes direct cells to grow and divide, while more yang genes inhibit growth. Researchers have discovered that women with breast cancer often have a preponderance of growth-enhancing genes, especially one gene known as the HER-2/neuoncogene located on chromosome 17. Scientists estimate that about 30 percent of women with breast cancer have as many as 50 of this more yin growth-enhancing gene. Normally only two are present. Moreover, researchers at the Cancer Institute in Tokyo hypothesize that the loss of a more yang growth-suppressing gene on chromosome 17 may also contribute to breast cancer. These findings suggest that breast cancer is a more yin condition, and that overintake of more extreme yin foods and beverages, including fats, influences the genetic structure of cells.

These characteristics suggest that breast and prostate cancer have opposite causes. Estrogen and other female hormones are more yin or expansive. They cause the female body to have a softer and more well-rounded form. Testosterone and other male hormones have an opposite, more yang quality. They cause the voice to deepen, behavior to be more aggressive, and growth of downward-growing facial and body hair to increase. Since testosterone (more yang) accelerates prostate cancer, and estrogen (more yin) helps neutralize it, the primary cause of prostate cancer is apparently an excess of yang factors in the body. Since breast cancer can be temporarily neutralized by more yang hormones and accelerated by more yin hormones, it has an opposite, more yin cause.

As we saw earlier, cancer develops over time as a result of the accumulation of excess in the body. Daily food is the source of the excess protein, fat, and mucous that promote the development of cancer. However, each food has a different quality and affects the body in a slightly different way. Some foods cause excess to accumulate primarily deep inside the body, while others accelerate the buildup of excess near the surface. The various ways in which dietary extremes affect our condition are due to the different yin and yang qualities of foods.

Macrobiotic Hope

My name is Magdaline Cronley and I live in the easternmost town on Long Island—Montauk—with my husband, Bob, and daughter Jennifer. I am forty-seven years old and was brought up on what is known as the "American diet." I consumed large quantities of meat, dairy products, sugar, frozen foods, and last, but not least, fast foods. I smoked cigarettes for over thirty years. Throughout my life I suffered with colds, flu, sinus problems, kidney infections, cysts, and weight problems.

In August 1984, I was diagnosed as having breast and lung cancer that had spread to various bones in my body. The prognosis was that I had two months to live as the cancer was deemed terminal and inoperable. I immediately began chemotherapy, which resulted in every hair on my body falling out and my not being able to "keep down" any food. When I wasn't vomiting, I was thinking about it. This way of life continued for a month, resulting in my body becoming weaker daily.

In September a woman named Joanne Kushi (formerly Joanne Collette), loaned my husband a copy of *The Cancer Prevention Diet* by Michio Kushi. That book was the ray of sunshine I had been waiting for. It became my Bible. I carried it around with me. It was on the night table next to my bed, in case I needed to look something up during the night. I started to see that if I ate the "American diet," I would feel worse and vomit because some of the additives in food and cosmetics were the same as those in my chemotherapy treatments. If I had a visitor who was, perhaps, wearing perfume or after-shave lotion containing these additives, I would say "hello" and have to excuse myself to go throw up.

As soon as I started to cook and eat miso soup, brown rice, and steamed vegetables, I began to feel better and stronger and the vomiting subsided. I started to cook in my wheelchair. Each day I was getting stronger. My doctor had wanted to give me two years of chemotherapy, which was twenty-two months longer than I was expected to live. He believed that without chemotherapy I would not survive. I continued chemotherapy for an additional six months, and prepared special dishes to rebuild my blood after each treatment.

I also had to deal with the cause of my cancer. I had to accept that smoking for thirty years had contributed to my lung cancer, and that eating a diet high in dairy products had most likely contributed to my breast cancer. Once I realized that I had helped my body get into this situation, I also realized that I could turn this illness into a blessing and allow God to heal me. I now had the ways and means to change my condition.

During January of 1985, I started to "call in well" for my chemotherapy treatments. I would feel so great that I didn't want to go for a treatment and spoil things, for example, by starting to vomit and losing my hair. (I had lost every hair on my body three times. I also grew back every hair three times with the help of good food.) My family went to Florida for a vacation and we walked on the beach, went into the salt water, ate good macrobiotic meals, and were thankful for what we had.

In March 1985 I went into the hospital for a blood transfusion after having been given too much chemotherapy. My doctor said that if I didn't have the transfusion, I would be in serious trouble if I came in contact with anyone carrying a germ that my immune system was unable to neutralize. In other words, my immune system was extremely weak. I realized that after the many x-rays, scans, and chemotherapy, my body had become toxic and had it not been for miso, sea vegetables, brown rice and vegetables, I probably would not have survived.

I started taking cooking classes and attending macrobiotic conferences and also went to the Kushi Institute in Becket, Massachusetts. I feel very fortunate to have been taught by the best teachers in the world. I realized that sharing had a great deal to do with my recovery. Our friend Joanne shared her knowledge and book with me, which resulted in my being able to heal myself. I was told that once you heal yourself, like it or not, you become a healer. I have since helped anyone who would listen and even, sometimes, those who weren't listening.

I teach cooking classes in our little hamlet of Montauk and nearby. To me, macrobiotics is not to be kept in a treasure chest, but is to be shared with whomever needs and wants to learn about it. Six years after my struggle with terminal cancer, I am alive and well, and thanking God for the opportunity to help others just as I was helped.

Source: Correspondence with Magdaline Cronley, August 7, 1990.

Yin and Yang in Food

Some foods have very condensed or contracting qualities, others are very expansive, and others are more balanced or centered. Meat, eggs, chicken, cheese, and other animal foods are very condensed. They are rich in sodium and other contractive minerals and contain hard saturated fat. Nutritionally, their main components are protein, fat, and minerals. These components correspond to the more yang physical structure of the body and are derived from animals that are ultimately nourished by plant foods. These components, therefore, represent the condensation of a tremendous volume of vegetable food. In addition, animal foods produce contraction in the body and are considered extremely yang. Eating a large volume of meat, eggs, cheese, or chicken produces constriction, stagnation, and tightening in the body. The saturated fat and cholesterol contained in animal foods are major causes of the buildup of fatty deposits that clog the arteries and other blood vessels, diminishing the free flow of blood and producing a condition of sluggishness or stagnation.

Vegetable foods are, on the whole, more yin or expansive. They are rich in potassium and other expansive elements, and, with few exceptions, contain a liquid form of unsaturated fat or oil, in contrast to the more yang saturated fat found in animal foods. Sugar, tropical fruits, spices, coffee, chocolate, nightshade vegetables, alcohol, and drugs or medications have more extreme yin or expansive effects. The simple sugars contained in many of these foods are used by the body primarily to generate quick energy. Simple sugars are rapidly absorbed into the bloodstream and are quickly metabolized. Rapid diffusion and decomposition are both yin tendencies. Many of these foods also contain plenty of water. Water dilutes substances, causing them to dissolve and melt. It produces swelling and expansion.

Foods such as whole cereal grains, beans, fresh local vegetables, sea vegetables, and temperate-climate fruits are, on the whole, more centrally balanced. They are not too yang or too yin, but have more neutral, harmonizing effects on the body. In Figure 5.1, foods are arranged according to yin and yang. The foods at the lower left generally have a greater degree of contracting force. Those appearing closer to the center (represented by intersecting lines of balance) have a more even balance of both forces, and those toward the upper right have a predominance of more yin, expanding energy.

There is a tremendous range of variation within each category of food. Animal foods are generally more condensed

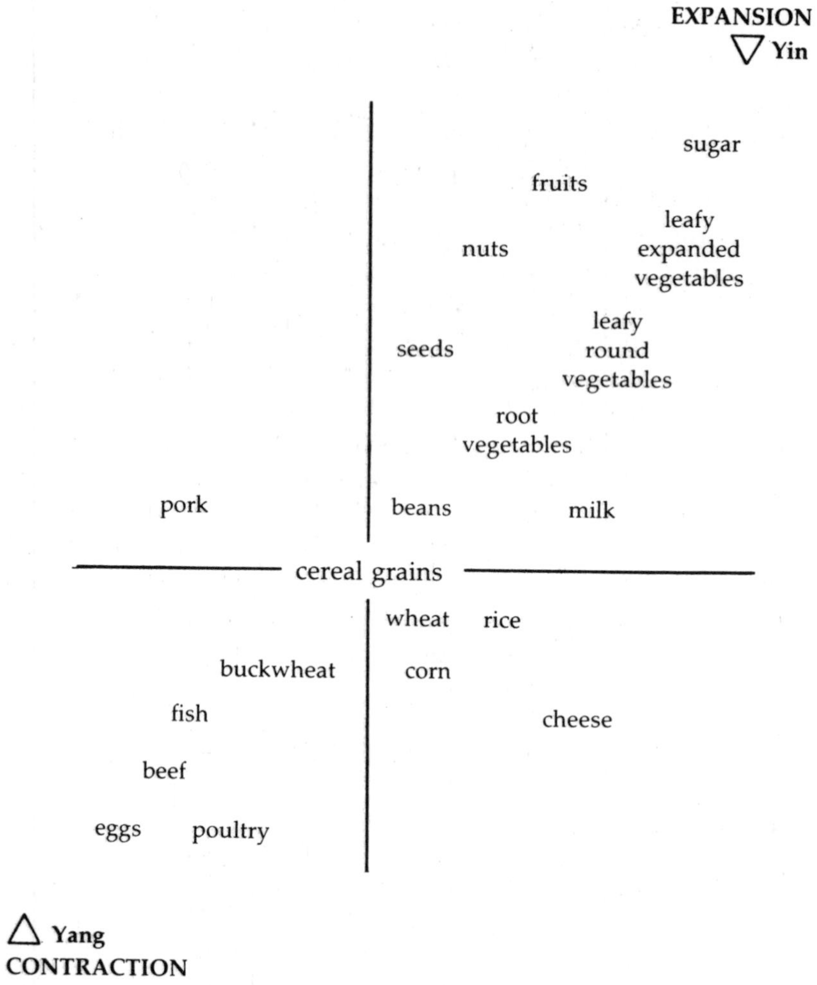

EXPANSION
▽ Yin

sugar

fruits

leafy
nuts   expanded
vegetables

leafy
seeds   round
vegetables

root
vegetables

pork   beans   milk

———————— cereal grains ————————

wheat   rice

buckwheat   corn

fish   cheese

beef

eggs   poultry

△ Yang
CONTRACTION

Figure 5.1   General Yin (▽) and Yang (△) Categorization of Foods

than grains or vegetables, but among the many types of animal foods, some are more contracting and others less so. Eggs, meat, and poultry, for example, have more extreme contracting energy than fish and other types of seafood. Among fish, those with red meat and blue skin are more extreme than white-meat varieties. Although dairy products come from an animal source, certain varieties — such as hard, salty cheeses — are more contracting, while others — such as yogurt, cottage cheese, milk, and ice cream—have a more expansive quality.

Although cereal grains are generally the most balanced of foods, a wide range of variation can be found among them; varieties such as buckwheat, millet, and winter wheat have more contracting effects, while summer wheat, barley, and corn are somewhat more expansive. Brown rice is generally in between, but again, this depends on the variety being considered. Short-grain rice, which is the most suitable variety for temperate climates, is generally the most balanced, followed by medium- and long-grain varieties, which are more appropriate for use in warmer areas.

Beans are generally more expansive than grains, but as with other categories of food, a wide range of variation exists among them. For example, certain varieties, such as azuki beans, chickpeas, and lentils, are smaller and lower in fat. They have more balanced energy than beans that are relatively larger or higher in fat, such as pinto, kidney, and lima beans.

Azuki beans provide a good example of the way in which climate and environment influence the quality of a food. Some azuki beans have a shiny surface and a deep maroon color. They are grown in mineral-rich volcanic soil on the northern Japanese island of Hokkaido, where the climate is similar to that of Maine. Other varieties have a somewhat faded color and a dull surface. They are grown in southern China in a warmer climate where the soil is less mineralized. Either variety is fine for regular use, but for the recovery of health, the mineral-rich Hokkaido beans, which are nutritionally superior, are preferred.

Soybeans have strong expanding energy, and this is reflected in their high fat and protein content. If their expanding qualities are not rebalanced through cooking or natural processing, the beans can be difficult to digest. One way to rebalance the energy in soybeans is to mix them with grains such as rice or barley, and age them with sea salt and enzymes to produce a product such as miso. When used properly, miso strengthens digestion, while making balanced proteins and beneficial enzymes available to the body. Among fermented soybean products, those such as miso and tamari soy sauce are aged for a longer period and have more concentrated energy, while those such as tofu and soy milk, which are quickly processed from the more expanded liquid portion of the bean, have more expanded energy.

Sea vegetables generally have more concentrated energy than most land vegetables, and this is reflected in their high mineral content. Those that grow closer to the shore or in warmer water are lighter and more expansive; those that grow in deeper, colder waters are more concentrated, as are those with a higher amount of minerals.

Vegetables generally have more expanding energy than grains or beans. Leafy green vegetables have more upward or expansive energy; round-shaped vegetables, such as cabbage, onion, and squash, are more evenly balanced; and root vegetables, such as carrots and burdock root, are more contracted. Along with shape, size, and direction of growth, place of origin is a key factor in creating a vegetable's energy quality. Vegetables such as tomato, potato, yams, avocado, eggplant, and peppers originated in South America or other tropical areas before being imported to Europe and North America. Compared to temperate varieties, like cabbage or kale, they have more extreme expanding energy, and, for this reason, it is better for people in temperate zones to avoid eating them.

In general, fruits have stronger expanding energy than vegetables. They are softer, sweeter, juicier, and are composed of more simple sugar. The place of origin also plays a decisive role in creating the quality of energy in each kind of fruit. Tropical or semi-tropical fruits—including pineapple, banana, kiwi, and citrus—have more extreme expanding energy than apples, pears, peaches, melons, and berries that grow in temperate zones. As with vegetables that originate in the tropics, these varieties of fruit have extreme expanding energy and are best avoided by persons who live in temperate zones.

Even more extreme energy can be found in concentrated sweeteners such as honey, maple syrup, and molasses, which are all very expansive, as are refined sugar and artificial sweeteners. Simple sugars, including those in fruits, are more yin or fragmented than centrally balanced complex carbohydrates such as those in whole grains, beans, and local vegetables. Other products that originate in the tropics—such as spices, coffee, chocolate, and carob—are also in the more extreme yin category, as is alcohol. But many drugs and medications, including aspirin and antibiotics, are even further out on the food spectrum. These products all have extremely expansive effects on the mind and body. The yin and yang characteristics of various products are presented in Table 5.2.

CLASSIFYING CANCERS

An example of the way in which extremes of yin or yang affect the body can be seen in the way they are discharged

Table 5.2   General Yin (∇) and Yang ($\triangle$) Classification of Food

Strong Yang Foods	More Balanced Foods	Strong Yin Foods
Refined salt	Unrefined white sea salt,	White rice, white flour
Eggs	miso, tamari soy sauce,	Frozen and canned foods
Meat	and other naturally	Tropical fruits and vegeta-
Hard cheese	salty seasonings	bles including those
Poultry	Tekka, gomashio, ume-	originating in the trop-
Lobster, crab,	boshi, and other natur-	ics—e.g., tomatoes and
and other	ally processed salty con-	potatoes
shellfish	diments	Milk, cream, yogurt, and
Red meat and	Low-fat, white-meat fish	ice cream
blue-skinned	Sea vegetables	Refined oils
fish	Whole cereal grains	Spices (pepper, curry, nut-
	Beans and bean products	meg, etc.)
	Root, round, and leafy	Aromatic and stimulant
	green vegetables from	beverages (coffee, black
	temperate climates	tea, mint tea, etc.)
	Fruits grown in temperate	Honey, sugar, and refined
	climates	sweeteners
	Nonaromatic, nonstimu-	Alcohol
	lant beverages	Foods containing chemi-
	Spring or well water	cals, preservatives, dyes,
	Naturally processed vege-	and pesticides
	table oils	Artificial sweeteners
	Brown rice syrup, barley	Drugs (marijuana, co-
	malt, and other natural	caine, etc., with a few
	grain-based sweeteners	exceptions)
	(when used moderately)	Medications (tranquiliz-
		ers, antibiotics, etc.,
		with some exceptions)

Source: The Macrobiotic Cancer Prevention Cookbook, Aveline Kushi and Wendy Esko (Avery Publishing Group, 1988).

through the skin. More yin simple sugars—including those in refined sugar, milk, and fruits—are often discharged in the form of freckles or large brown age spots. These markings are formed by melanin, a dark brown pigment produced by more yin branch-shaped cells in the epidermis. More yang animal foods produce a different kind of skin marking. Rather than causing numerous spots to appear over the surface of the body, animal foods often cause moles—hard, condensed growths—to appear on the skin.

The fats and other forms of excess contained in animal foods tend to gather deep inside the body—in the blood vessels, including those surrounding the heart; in organs such as the ovaries and pancreas; in the inner regions of the brain; and in the bones. Hard animal fats also accumulate in the lower body, for example, in the prostate, colon, and rectum. The fats and other forms of excess that are produced by milk, sugar, chocolate, and other simple carbohydrates tend to gather toward the upper regions of the body, including the breasts, or in peripheral areas such as the skin or outer regions of the brain. Either type of accumulation can promote the development of cancer.

Returning to our example of breast and prostate cancer, we can see that prostate cancer develops deep within the body in a small, compact gland, and is promoted by the overconsumption of meat, cheese, chicken, eggs, and other yang extremes. (These foods also accelerate production of testosterone.) Breast cancer develops near the periphery of the body in the more expanded, soft tissue of the breasts, and is promoted by excess consumption of milk, ice cream, soft cheese, chocolate, refined sugar, and other yin extremes. (These foods also promote the secretion of estrogen.)

Estrogen, which plays a role in the growth of breast tumors, is secreted not only in the ovaries, but in more yin fat cells. Women who are obese have higher levels of estrogen than women who are thin, and also have a greater risk of breast cancer after menopause. Moreover, researchers at the Naylor Dana Institute in Valhalla, New York, have discovered that when women switch to a diet low in fat (20 percent of total calories) their estrogen levels rapidly decline by 20 percent, showing that fat intake has a definite influence on cancer. The production of estrogen is promoted especially by the overconsumption of milk, ice cream, butter, and other high-fat foods, as well as by chocolate, refined sugar, and other extremely yin foods and beverages.

Cancers of the upper digestive tract, including those in the stomach and esophagus, are accelerated by the overconsumption of yin extremes. Cancers of the lower digestive tract, including colo-rectal cancer, are promoted primarily by an excessive intake of yang extremes. That explains why the Japanese have a high rate of stomach cancer and a low rate of colon cancer, and why Americans experience the opposite incidence: a low rate of stomach cancer and a high rate of colon cancer. The Japanese tend to develop more stomach cancers because they eat a large volume of sugar, chemicals, and more yin, chemically grown and treated white rice. The consumption of alcohol and a lack of chewing contribute to the development of an overacid condition in the stomach that can promote the eventual development of cancer. Americans develop more colon cancers primarily because of their high intake of meat, eggs, cheese, and other extreme yang animal foods. Of course, yin and yang foods are always eaten in combination. But certain people eat a larger volume of one, while some eat a larger volume of the other, and these differences influence the types of cancer they develop.

Skin cancer, which develops at the periphery of the body, is promoted by the overconsumption of more yin foods and beverages, while bone cancer, which develops deeper inside, is accelerated by the consumption of more yang dietary extremes. Leukemia, a disease of the blood, is characterized by a decrease in the number of red blood cells together with a dramatic increase in the number of white blood cells. Leukemia patients may have as many as one million white blood cells per cubic mm of blood instead of the normal 5,000 to 6,000.

White blood cells are more yin than red blood cells. Red blood cells are generally smaller and more compact, while white blood cells are larger. An increase in the number of white blood cells indicates an overly yin condition in the blood and in the body as a whole. This condition is promoted by overconsumption of sugar, soft drinks, ice cream, milk, chemicals, and other yin extremes. At the same time, a decrease in the number of red blood cells reflects a lack of minerals and other more yang factors in the diet.

Meat Consumption and Colon Cancer

In a study conducted at Brigham and Women's Hospital in Boston and released in December 1990, persons who eat beef, pork, or lamb every day were found to be twice as likely to get colon cancer as those who avoid red meat. The study was conducted on 88,751 women, and provides some of the strongest evidence yet that a diet high in red meat contributes to this type of cancer.

The study was based on a follow-up of the health and eating habits of nurses throughout the United States during the period from 1980 to 1986. The researchers discovered that women who ate pork, beef, or lamb as a main dish every day were two-and-a-half times more likely to develop colon cancer than those who ate these foods less than once a month. Processed meats were significantly associated with a higher risk of colon cancer. Commenting on the results, Dr. Walter C. Willet, the director of the study said, "Moderate red meat intake is certainly better than large amounts, but it's quite possible that no red meat intake is even better."

Hodgkin's disease and lymphosarcoma are also more yin forms of cancer. In Hodgkin's disease, the lymph nodes and spleen become inflammed; in lymphosarcoma, tumors form in the lymphoid tissue and the lymphatic organs become swollen. As in leukemia, both diseases involve an increase in the number of white blood cells.

Like the opposite poles of a magnet, yin and yang attract one another. The more extreme the diet becomes at one end of the food spectrum, the more we require opposite extremes to make balance. In this century, rising intakes of meat and poultry (yang foods) have required progressively more powerful forms of yin to make balance. Sugar, chocolate, coffee, nightshade vegetables, spices, and tropical fruits are commonly used today. But beyond these, many people turn to the frequent consumption of alcohol, or to drugs, which are even more extreme. In some cases, the combination of both ex-

CHRONIC MYELOCYTIC LEUKEMIA

Healing Cancer with Love

My mother and I were very close. When she was diagnosed with colon cancer in 1982, I thought nothing worse could happen. Then, when she died in 1984, at the age of 49, my life was rocked to the core. Her illness and death, ironically, set me on the path I follow today.

I watched as conventional methods of treatment hastened her deterioration. Watching her suffer more with each treatment strengthened my conviction to seek out alternative treatments should I ever find myself in a similar situation. I had absolutely no idea what that meant, but I knew that I could never go through a similar ordeal. Interestingly, one of her doctors mentioned macrobiotics to me, but it was too late for her, and I forgot all about it.

My maternal family history is checkered with diabetes, cancer, and anemia, so it was no surprise when, as a child, I was diagnosed with Mediterranean Anemia. Every female member of my family was plagued with this disease.

Throughout my teenage years, I seemed relatively healthy, but always had the hardest time healing cuts and scratches. Bruises seemed to appear from nowhere. Stamina was always a problem as well. My menstrual cycle was irregular and so doctors began hormone treatments that would last for over 15 years.

At the age of 14, I decided to become a vegetarian (whatever that means). I continued to eat lots of dairy, sugar, and refined foods. After my mother died, my fatigue worsened. I thought it was just an accumulation of exhaustion from over two years of taking care of her and dealing with my grief. I felt drained all the time. As the months after her death wore on, it seemed that my condition worsened—bruises were appearing everywhere; I felt as though my insides were on fire.

Finally, after five months of living in this manner, I decided that a fresh start was what I needed. So I packed up and left Florida and moved north to Philadelphia. As I settled into my new surroundings, my health continued to worsen. Bruises appeared from nowhere; minor scratches became infected and would not heal; and I was exhausted. I finally decided to see a doctor, who, after a battery of tests, referred me to a hemotologist/oncologist. I was put through every test they could think of, after which they came up with the diagnosis of chronic myelocytic leukemia.

So here I was, twenty-seven years old, sitting in a room with five hemotologists recounting my options—as they saw them. Seeing a lymphocyte count as high as mine, they really did not see a sunny future for me. However, they did want to propose experimental chemotherapy and a possible bone marrow transplant. When I questioned them as to a time frame, their response was not encouraging—three months to live with no treatment, and six months to a year with treatment. It seemed to me that the only guarantee I could get from them was that I would lose my hair and feel lousy for the time I had left. All I could think of was what my mother went through. I said I needed a few days to digest all of this. I knew I would never go back there.

For about a week, I walked around in a daze. Here I was, faced with this crisis, in a new city, with nowhere to turn. Finally I spoke to a friend at work and told him everything. I told him that my plan was to return to Europe and live there until the end came. He suggested that before I did anything quite that drastic, I meet a friend of his who ate this strange diet that was supposed to help people recover from diseases like cancer. I figured I had nothing to lose and agreed.

That weekend I was introduced to Robert Pirello, who had been practicing macrobiotics for eight years, and my life was changed forever.

Bob was great. He listened to all my fears and finally agreed to help me as much as he could. The next day, we went shopping. I watched as Bob loaded up my cart with all these unfamiliar foods. I couldn't even pronounce the names—I was going to cook and eat them? But, then again, I thought, I had always loved a challenge. What bigger challenge than seeing if I could heal my own illness?

We went back to my apartment and Bob cleaned out my cupboards—throwing away all the old foods and replacing them with this new food. As I watched, I began to get really scared—a challenge was one thing, but this was my life. If I messed this up, there were no second chances. As Bob left, he handed me *The Cancer Prevention Diet* by Michio Kushi, telling me to read and cook. I read all night.

We met for lunch every day. Bob brought rice balls or leftovers from his own dinner. (Although I was a great conventional cook, my macrobiotic cooking was terrible then.) We talked and talked and I read and read. After a few weeks, I had lost weight and had more energy. Then I had a blood test—my lymphocyte count had worsened. Now I was scared. Even macrobiotics wasn't working. I felt hopeless. But, with Bob's encouragement, I persevered. I began to cook in earnest. It suddenly occurred to me that only I could make me well. Bob wanted me to meet with a macrobiotic teacher. I refused. I needed to do this on my own; a teacher would only be another crutch—someone else to take responsibility for me. *I needed to do this for me.*

I continued to cook and eat, and things started to improve. Even my blood tests were beginning to reverse—ever so slightly. But that was enough to give me hope. I thought the worst was over. God, we can be so naive sometimes. To think that I could change my life so drastically with no "payback" was insane. But maybe it's better to be ignorant. The discharging began full force. First, the diarrhea that lasted a couple of weeks. I was so depleted, I thought I would never survive.

Then my skin began to break out. The itching and erupting spread until I was completely covered with a rash. When that cleared (after eight weeks), I was left with a face full of pimples that would plague me for almost two years. Menstrual problems including an ovarian cyst developed. Hip baths and bancha tea douches solved that problem, only to be replaced by more discharging.

And so it went. Although the discharge was always unpleasant and almost impossible to bear, I knew I was improving. Each blood test revealed an improvement in my white cell count. The doctors were amazed. They called it "spontaneous regression" and said it was very rare—and could reverse at any time. I now know differently. Thirteen months after my practice of macrobiotics began, my white cell count was declared within normal range, where it has remained for almost seven years now.

And what did the doctors have to say? Well, they said that spontaneous regression never yielded results like these, so this miraculous improvement had to be the result of something else. I then told them about macrobiotics. They called it "voodoo" and said it had nothing to do with my recovery. When I persisted, they said that I was probably misdiagnosed in the first place. I was blind with rage. I knew what I had just been through. Misdiagnosed? I was appalled at their arrogance and lack of vision. I left—and have never returned.

When I began my practice of macrobiotics, I was going to eat and get well. The philosophy was of little interest to me. But as my health improved, so did my clarity and judgment. Even now, it seems as though the fog continues to disperse each day, and I wonder how I could have been blind to the order of the universe for so much of my life.

It is hard for me to remember the person I was before macrobiotics. Bob and I married and have created a wonderful life together. My gratitude to him is boundless—he was my teacher and my support system through the darkest times. We are the publishers of a newsletter—*MacroNews*—that reaches many people in the Philadelphia area and around the world, and is committed to sharing what we know to be the natural order. I work as a macrobiotic cook in a natural foods store and have begun to conduct cooking classes in our home. (Yes, my cooking has improved dramatically since the beginning) I feel strong and my health continues to improve. Life is a wonder to me now.

People seem amazed when I tell them that cancer was the best thing to ever happen to me. Yet, without that trial, I would never have met my wonderful husband to whom I owe my very life. I would never have learned what true responsibility for oneself can mean. And chances are, I would have never discovered this way of life that has the potential of changing our entire civilization into what it was meant to be.

Source: "Macrobiotics: Getting Started," by Christina Pirello, *MacroNews*, Jan./Feb. 1990.

tremes promotes the development of cancer; melanoma is an example of this type of cancer.

Melanoma usually appears initially on an existing mole and spreads quickly through the lymph or blood to the lungs, liver, brain, intestines, reproductive organs, or other sites. The overconsumption of yin extremes, including sugar, fats and oils and milk, promotes the tendency of the cancer to appear at the surface of the body. Overconsumption of chicken, cheese, eggs, and other more yang animal foods accelerates the tendency for the cancer to spread and develop internally.

To summarize, certain cancers are promoted by the overconsumption of extremely yin foods, others are promoted by too many yang extremes, while others result from an excess of both extremes. In Table 5.3, we classify common varieties of cancer according to yin and yang.

CANCER PROMOTERS, CANCER INHIBITORS

Yin and yang help clarify the role that foods have in promoting or inhibiting cancer. For example, epidemiological studies have found that the incidence of colon cancer is higher in the

Table 5.3 General Yin(∇) and Yang($\triangle$) Classification of Cancer Sites

Extreme Yin Cancer Site	Extreme Yang Cancer Site	Combined Yin and Yang Cancer Site
Breast	Colon	Lung
Stomach	Prostate	Bladder
Skin	Rectum	Uterus
Mouth (except tongue)	Ovary	Kidney
Esophagus	Bone	Spleen
Leukemia	Pancreas	Melanoma
Hodgkin's Disease	Brain (inner regions)	Tongue
Brain (outer regions)		

United States and other countries where the consumption of meat and saturated fat (yang) is high, and where the consumption of fiber is low. In December 1986, the *New England Journal of Medicine* added to the evidence with a report on a study in which men with high cholesterol levels were found to be 60 percent more likely to develop colon cancer than those with normal cholesterol levels. (Another study found a relationship between high cholesterol and colon polyps that often turn cancerous.) Meat, eggs, dairy foods, and other animal products are the chief sources of saturated fat and cholesterol in the modern diet.

On the other hand, populations that consume less animal food and more cereal grains and other plant fibers (yin) have much lower rates of colon cancer. As we have seen, the over-consumption of too many strong yang animal foods promotes the development of cancer in the lower digestive tract, especially colo-rectal cancer. Plant fibers, which are relatively more yin, offset this tendency and thereby have a protective effect. Vegetable fibers disperse potentially harmful accumulations of fat and mucus in the intestines. They help prevent the sluggishness or stagnation that results from consuming too many animal foods.

In a similar way, leafy green and orange-yellow vegetables, which are high in beta-carotene, help protect against lung cancer. Lung cancer is promoted by an excessive consumption of extremes of both yin and yang, especially meat, eggs, cheese, and other high-fat animal foods, and sugar, chemicals, and refined foods. Vegetable foods help slow the buildup of animal fats that underlie the development of cancer.

Several years ago it was discovered that the fat and protein molecules contained in charcoal grilled meat or fish can promote cancer. However, people have eaten foods such as grilled sardines, fish, or meat for thousands of years, yet rarely developed cancer. Traditionally, these foods were eaten together with plenty of fresh green vegetables, creating a complementary balance that prevented cancer from developing. Again, the cancer-causing potential of these extreme yang foods is neutralized or offset by the yin qualities contained in plant foods.

Some people believe that the sun causes skin cancer. However, of itself, the sun is not the cause of this disease. Many people are able to spend long periods of time in the sun and never develop skin cancer. The predisposition to this cancer comes from our underlying condition, and this is determined by our dietary habits. The consumption of milk, cheese, and other animal fats, and sugar, soft drinks, chemicalized food, and other yin extremes provides the underlying basis for skin cancer to develop. The sun, a more yang influence, attracts yin excess in the body and causes it to be discharged through the skin. If the volume of excess is moderate, it produces skin markings such as freckles and aging spots. These markings represent the discharge of excess sugar and simple carbohydrates. If the amount of excess in the body is great, the accumulation of excess can lead to the cell changes that promote cancer. However, the source of excess is diet, not the sun.

The foods in the macrobiotic diet come primarily from the more centrally balanced category. When eaten in the proper proportions, they help neutralize or offset the effects of dietary extremes. A naturally balanced diet keeps the body free of toxic buildup, and helps the body naturally discharge accumulations of excess. In the next chapter, we look more closely at the foods in the standard macrobiotic diet and at their role in inhibiting cancer and promoting health.

6

Foods That
Promote Health

The healing power of the standard macrobiotic diet derives
from its overall reliance on centrally balanced foods, and not
from the isolated effects of any one particular food or chemical compound. At the same time, researchers have discovered
that the primary categories of food in the standard macrobiotic diet (whole grains, beans and bean products, fresh local vegetables, and sea vegetables) have specific properties
that inhibit cancer. Evidence is now accumulating that primary macrobiotic foods not only prevent cancer from developing, but also slow or inhibit its development. Some of the
possible cancer-inhibiting substances found in macrobiotic
foods are shown in Table 6.1.

In this chapter, we present a more elaborate list of foods
that are included in the macrobiotic diet, and mention some
of the scientific research linking these primary foods to reduced cancer risk. Also presented are general guidelines for
adopting the standard macrobiotic diet for the recovery of
health. (More specific recommendations are presented in *The
Cancer Prevention Diet* listed in Recommended Reading on
page 161. Readers who would like more detailed advice are
encouraged to refer to this book.) These guidelines are not
substitutes for qualified medical care. Persons with serious ill-

Table 6.1   Possible Cancer-Inhibiting Substances in Basic Macrobiotic Foods

Food	Cancer-Inhibiting Factors
Whole grains	Fiber, protease inhibitors
Beans and bean products	Fiber, protease inhibitors
Orange-yellow vegetables	Beta-carotene and other carotenoid pigments, fiber
Green leafy vegetables	Beta-carotene and other carotenoid pigments, chlorophyll, fiber
Cruciferous vegetables	Indoles, dithiolthiones, glucosinolates, carotenoids, chlorophyll, fiber
Sea vegetables	Fiber, chlorophyll, fucoidan

ness are, of course, advised to consult with a qualified medical or nutritional professional at the earliest opportunity.

As we saw in Chapter 2, the recommended percentages of foods in the standard macrobiotic diet are for an entire day, and are calculated by volume and not by weight. It isn't necessary to include all of these categories at every meal, nor to include all of these foods at once when beginning macrobiotics. Start with the basic staples and broaden your selection as you familiarize yourself with these new foods. Breakfast, for example, is often more simple, consisting of a whole grain porridge, miso soup, and a few basic side dishes; lunch and dinner can be more elaborate. However, it is important to have whole grains as your main food at each meal and to have adequate variety in your daily diet as a whole.

The recipes in *The Macrobiotic Cancer Prevention Cookbook* and other cookbooks listed at the end of this chapter can help you get started with a wide range of foods and translate these guidelines into delicious and nourishing meals.

Principal foods are normally eaten daily and include whole grains, beans and bean products, vegetables, and sea vegetables. Low-fat white-meat fish, seasonal fruits, natural desserts, nuts, seeds, natural sweeteners, and other supplementary foods are eaten less often. Condiments, pickles, snacks, seasonings, and beverages can be used daily but in smaller quantities than principal foods. "Occasional use" foods may be consumed an average of two or three times per week, while "infrequent use" foods should not be consumed more than two or three times per month.

The guidelines that follow are broad and flexible. The standard macrobiotic way of eating offers an incredible variety of foods and cooking methods to choose from. These guidelines form the basis for the natural recovery of health and the prevention of illness, and can be applied when selecting the highest quality natural foods for daily meals.

WHOLE CEREAL GRAINS

Whole cereal grains are the staff of life and an essential part of a balanced diet. They constitute up to 50 to 60 percent of the standard macrobiotic diet. Below is a list of the whole grains and grain products that are frequently included:

Regular Use

Barley
Buckwheat
Corn
Medium grain brown
  rice (in warmer areas
  or seasons)
Millet

Pearl barley (hato mugi)
Rye
Short grain brown rice
Whole oats
Whole wheat berries
Other traditionally used
  whole grains

Occasional Use

Corn grits
Corn meal
Couscous
Cracked wheat
  (bulghur)
Long grain brown rice
Mochi (a cake made
  from pounded sweet
  brown rice)

Rolled oats
Rye, wheat, rice and
  other whole grain
  flakes
Steel cut oats
Sweet brown rice
Other traditionally
  used whole grain
  products

Occasional Use Flour Products

Fu	Unyeasted whole rye bread
Seitan	Unyeasted whole wheat
Soba (buckwheat)	bread
noodles	Whole wheat noodles
Somen (thin wheat)	Other whole grain products
noodles	that were used
Udon (wheat) noodles	traditionally

Cooked whole grains are preferable to flour products or to cracked or rolled grains because of their easier digestibility. In general, it is better to keep the intake of flour products — or cracked or rolled grains — to less than 15 to 20 percent of your daily consumption of whole grains.

Cancer-Inhibiting Properties

A wide variety of studies show that, as a part of a balanced diet, whole grains, which are high in fiber and bran, protect against nearly all forms of cancer. For example, in 1981, Pelayo Correa, a researcher at the Louisiana State University Medical Center, reported a worldwide association between low death rates from cancer of the breast, colon, and prostate and a high per capita consumption of rice, sweet corn (maize), and beans. At present, thirty-two worldwide studies have associated consumption of high-fiber grains and grain products with lowered rates of colon cancer. Laboratory studies also show that cereal grains have a cancer-protective effect. For example, rice bran, the outer coating of brown rice, has been shown in animal experiments to reduce the incidence of cancer in the large intestine. Japanese scientists have isolated several substances in rice bran that have cancer-inhibiting properties, and have found that these substances suppressed the growth of solid tumors in mice.

The Senate Select Committee's report *Dietary Goals for the United States*, the National Academy of Sciences' report *Diet, Nutrition and Cancer*, the dietary guidelines of the American Cancer Society, and many others call for substantial increases in the consumption of whole grains.

Brown rice, barley, wheat, oats, rye, corn, and other whole

grains contain compounds known as protease inhibitors that are believed to suppress the action of proteases, enzymes suspected of promoting cancer. Protease inhibitors may also interfere with the activity of oncogenes, which, under certain circumstances, are thought to stimulate normal cells to turn cancerous.

Researchers at the Harvard School of Public Health have experimented with protease inhibitors and have found that they prevent cells damaged by carcinogens from turning cancerous, and cause carcinogen-damaged cells to return to normal. According to Dr. Walter Troll, a professor of environmental medicine at New York University who has done extensive research on protease inhibitors, eating foods high in these substances can inhibit cancer development even in its later stages.

General Guidelines

For the improvement of health, it is best to temporarily limit or avoid eating baked flour products such as cookies, muffins, crackers, chapatis, etc., even when they are made from whole grain flours. However, natural unyeasted whole grain sourdough bread can be eaten when craved, usually several times per week; whole wheat noodles (udon) can also be included several times per week, preferably in soup or broth. (Persons who have had surgery within the past two years are advised to temporarily avoid buckwheat noodles [soba] and whole buckwheat [kasha].) Oatmeal made from rolled or cut oats is also best avoided as are other rolled, milled, or partially refined grains or grain products until the condition improves.

Short grain brown rice is recommended as the primary grain for daily consumption, and pressure cooking is the preferred method for preparing brown rice in a temperate climate. For variety, brown rice can be cooked with grains such as millet, barley, pearl barley (hato mugi), and wheat berries, or with azuki or other beans. These ingredients can be cooked in the same dish, using, for example, 80-85 percent brown rice and 15-20 percent of these other ingredients. Porridge made from leftover brown rice and other whole grains can be eaten as a hot breakfast cereal. Simply add water to leftover grains and reheat. Corn on the cob, fresh and in season, can also be eaten several times per week, without butter.

SOUPS

Soups comprise about five percent of the standard macrobiotic diet. For most people, that averages out to about one or two cups or small bowls per day. A wide variety of ingredients, including vegetables, grains, beans, sea vegetables, noodles, tofu, tempeh, and, occasionally, white-meat fish are wonderful in soups. Soups are delicious when moderately seasoned with either miso, tamari soy sauce, sea salt, umeboshi plum or paste, or occasional ginger.

Soups can be made thick and rich, or as simple clear broths. Vegetable, grain, or bean stews can also be enjoyed, while a variety of garnishes, such as scallions, parsley, and nori sea vegetable may be used to enhance the appearance and flavor of soups.

Light miso soup, with vegetables and wakame or kombu, is recommended daily—on average, one small bowl or cup per day. Mugi (barley) miso is the best for regular consumption, followed by soybean (hatcho) miso. A second cup or bowl of soup may also be enjoyed, preferably mildly seasoned with tamari soy sauce or sea salt. Other healthful varieties of soup include:

> Bean and vegetable   Puréed squash and
>   soups   other vegetable soups
>   Grain and vegetable soups

Cancer-Inhibiting Properties

Practically all of the ingredients commonly used in miso and other macrobiotic soups have cancer-inhibiting properties. Miso itself is made from naturally fermented soybeans and grains, which contain fiber and high levels of protease inhibitors. Miso soup frequently includes orange-yellow and green leafy vegetables, which are high in beta-carotene, as well as cabbage, cauliflower, turnips, and other cruciferous vegeta-

"Avoid Dying of Cancer"

Back in 1982 when I was 75, I had been going to an internist every year for a complete physical check-up. This included a sigmoidoscope of the colon but, for some reason, did not include the Hemoccult II slide test, which checks the feces for blood. In March of 1982, several months after my last examination, I consulted my internist again regarding pain in the abdomen and he prescribed a tranquilizer for "gas."

My guardian angel must have been looking out for me when I saw a newspaper write-up about a course entitled "Avoid Dying of Cancer—Now or Later" conducted once a year at Ohio State University. While it is attended primarily by approximately 300 medical and nursing students, senior citizens can attend without charge. Included in the course is voluntary testing of the feces for blood by the Hemoccult II slide method. In the course I learned that everyone over 50 years of age should have such a check once a year. The test can be done at home in privacy.

My test was positive whereupon I had a barium enema that showed a tumor in the colon. It was removed without a colostomy. One year later, the results of a liver CAT scan prompted me to investigate the macrobiotic diet. I learned of it from a TV newscast that told how Dr. Anthony Sattilaro had picked up two hitchhikers and learned of the diet.

I attended the Macrobiotic Way of Life Seminar in Boston to learn about cooking, home care, and macrobiotic principles. Since then I have attended four of the very beneficial macrobiotic summer conferences presented in the Berkshires. For a year after going on the diet, I was given a medical check-up every three months. Now I only have to go in once a year. With the support of my wife, Margaret, many changes were made in lifestyle, the food we purchase, the way it is prepared, how we eat, and in other aspects. I increased my amount of exercise. As a result, I experienced weight control from a lowered fat intake. My cholesterol went from 219 to 137, and I feel physically and mentally more alert and good enough to take several trips a year. My CEA levels are well within the normal range and there is no sign of a recurrence of the cancer.

Source: Correspondence with Cecil O. Dudley, Columbus, Ohio, August 1990.

bles containing substances called indoles. As discussed below, these substances are now considered to have a wide range of anti-cancer effects. Moreover, shiitake mushrooms, also noted for their cancer-inhibiting properties (see below), are often added to miso soup, as are wakame, kombu, and other sea vegetables that have also been discovered to inhibit the development of tumors.

In 1981 Japan's National Cancer Center reported that people who eat miso soup daily are 33 percent less likely to develop stomach cancer and have 19 percent less cancer at other sites than those who never eat miso soup. The 13-year study, involving about 265,000 men and women over 40, also found that those who never ate miso soup had a 43 percent higher death rate from coronary heart disease than those who consumed miso soup daily. Those who abstained from miso also had 29 percent more fatal strokes, 3.5 times more deaths resulting from high blood pressure, and higher mortality from all other causes.

General Guidelines

Miso is processed with natural sea salt, so use it in moderation. Miso soup should have a mild flavor and not be too salty. It can be eaten once and sometimes twice per day. Change the recipe often. Other soups—including grain, bean, and vegetable soups—can also be eaten for variety and enjoyment.

VEGETABLES

Roughly one quarter to one third (25 to 30 percent) of daily intake can include vegetables. Nature provides an incredible variety of fresh local vegetables to choose from. Available vegetables include:

Regular Use

Acorn squash	Hubbard squash
Bok choy	Jinenjo
Broccoli	Kale

Brussels sprouts
Burdock
Butternut squash
Cabbage
Carrots
Carrot tops
Cauliflower
Chinese cabbage
Collard greens
Daikon
Daikon greens
Dandelion greens
Dandelion roots
Hokkaido pumpkin

Leeks
Lotus root
Mustard greens
Onions
Parsley
Parsnip
Pumpkin
Radish
Red cabbage
Rutabaga
Scallions
Turnip
Turnip greens
Watercress

Occasional Use

Celery
Chives
Coltsfoot
Cucumber
Endive
Escarole
Green beans
Green peas
Iceberg lettuce
Jerusalem artichoke
Kohlrabi

Lambs-quarters
Mushrooms
Pattypan squash
Romaine lettuce
Salsify
Shiitake mushrooms
Snap beans
Snow peas
Sprouts
Summer squash
Wax beans

Avoid (for Optimal Health)

Artichoke
Bamboo shoots
Beets
Curly dock
Eggplant
Fennel
Ferns
Ginseng
Green/red pepper
New Zealand
  spinach
Okra

Plaintain
Potato
Purslane
Shepherd's-purse
Sorrel
Spinach
Sweet potato
Swiss chard
Taro (albi) potato
Tomato
Yams
Zucchini

Vegetables can be served in soups, or with grains, beans, or sea vegetables. They can also be used in making rice rolls (homemade sushi), served with noodles or pasta, cooked with fish, or served alone. The most common methods for cooking vegetables include boiling, steaming, pressing, sautéing (both waterless and with oil), and pickling. A variety of natural seasonings, including miso, tamari soy sauce, sea salt, and brown rice vinegar or umeboshi vinegar are recommended in vegetable cookery. Vegetables from tropical climates are not recommended for use in the temperate zones, neither are nightshade vegetables such as tomatoes, potatoes and eggplant. Three to five vegetable side dishes can be prepared daily to ensure adequate variety.

Cancer-Inhibiting Properties

A wide range of studies have shown that regular intake of cooked vegetables, especially leafy greens and orange-yellow vegetables, helps protect against cancer. Shiitake mushrooms, which are used often in miso and other soups and in a variety of macrobiotic dishes, have also been noted for their cancer-inhibiting properties. In 1970 Japanese scientists at the National Cancer Center Research Institute reported that shiitake mushrooms had a strong anti-tumor effect. In experiments with mice, polysaccharide preparations from various natural sources, including the shiitake mushroom commonly available in Tokyo markets, markedly inhibited the growth of induced sarcomas, resulting in almost complete regression of tumors with no apparent toxicity.

In studies conducted in 1960 by Dr. Kenneth Cochoran of the University of Michigan, shiitake mushrooms were found to contain a strong antiviral substance that strengthened immune response. Researchers now theorize that the shiitake mushroom stimulates the body's production of interferon, an immune substance that counteracts viruses and cancer.

Cruciferous vegetables, including cabbage, Brussels sprouts, broccoli, cauliflower, and turnips, are recommended for frequent or daily use in the macrobiotic diet. These vegetables are also recognized for their cancer-inhibiting properties. In a study conducted in the 1970s by Dr. Saxon Graham,

Naturally Sweet Vegetables

Naturally sweet vegetables, such as cabbage, squash, carrots, onions, and parsnips, provide a readily available source of complex carbohydrates that can help reduce the symptoms of hypoglycemia, including fatigue, anxiety, depression, and an overpowering craving for sugar and other sweets. They may be eaten regularly in the diet, or taken in the more concentrated form of sweet vegetable drink. To prepare this special drink, cut equal amounts of carrots, squash (select those with an orange color on the inside), onions, and green cabbage into very fine pieces. Place the cut vegetables in a pot with four times as much water, cover, and bring to a boil. Reduce the flame to low and simmer for fifteen to twenty minutes. Remove from the stove and strain the liquid through a fine mesh strainer into a large glass jar. The leftover vegetable pieces can be used in soups, stews, or other dishes.

The strained liquid—or "sweet vegetable drink"—can be stored in the refrigerator for several days. One or two cups can be taken daily or several times per week depending on the severity of the condition. Sweet vegetable drink may be continued for a month or so or until the symptoms of hypoglycemia improve. To serve, heat in a saucepan until warm, or allow it to set for several minutes until it becomes room temperature.

chaiman of social and preventive medicine at the State University of New York, the diets of 256 men with cancer of the colon were compared to those of 783 men who did not have cancer. The men who ate the most cabbage, Brussels sprouts, broccoli, turnips, cauliflower, and other vegetables were found to have the lowest rates of cancer. The researchers discovered that the more of these vegetables eaten, the greater the protective effect. Among the vegetables studied, cabbage was found to have the most beneficial effect: eating cabbage more than once a week reduced the risk of colon cancer by two-thirds.

Lee Wattenberg, M.D., of the University of Minnesota Medical School investigated cruciferous vegetables and, in a 1978 article in *Cancer Research*, reported that they contained chemicals known as indoles. Along with other minor constituents, including chlorophyll, carotenoids, dithiolthiones, and glucosinolates, indoles are believed to inhibit the various stages of cancer formation. For example, researchers at Johns Hopkins University now consider dithiolthiones to be potent anti-cancer agents. According to Dr. Wattenberg, eating foods high in these substances strengthens the body's detoxification system, or ability to discharge toxic excess. Epidemiological studies conducted in the United States, Japan, Israel, Greece, and Norway have shown that people who eat a higher proportion of cruciferous vegetables have lower rates of colon cancer. These vegetables are also associated with lower rates of lung, esophagus, larynx, prostate, bladder, and rectal cancer.

Beta-carotene, and other carotenoid pigments found in orange-yellow and dark leafy green vegetables, have also been shown to have cancer-inhibiting effects. A 1981 Chicago study found that regular consumption of foods containing beta-carotene (a precursor to vitamin A) protected against lung cancer. Over a period of 19 years, 1,954 men at a Western Electric plant were monitored, and those who regularly ate carrots, broccoli, kale, Chinese cabbage, and other carotene-rich foods had significantly lower lung cancer rates than did the controls. The study, published in *The Lancet*, reported that men with the lowest consumption of beta-carotene foods had a seven times greater risk of lung cancer than men with the highest intakes. In the laboratory, beta-carotene was found to prevent skin cancer from developing in animals exposed to ultraviolet light, and to inhibit both the formation and growth of tumors. Researchers have also identified other carotenoid pigments in these vegetables that are believed to inhibit the development of cancer.

General Guidelines

Vegetables in the "Regular Use" column may be eaten daily, while those in the "Occasional Use" column may be eaten once or twice per week on average. In certain cases, especially when a person feels weak or has impaired digestion, it may be necessary to temporarily avoid the intake of raw salad or vegetables. Instead, dishes such as quickly boiled (blanched) salad, pressed salad, and steamed greens can be eaten daily or often. In normal circumstances, a small amount of high quality sesame oil can be used about three times per week in sautéing vegetables and other foods; however, when a large volume of high-fat animal foods has been recently consumed, it may be necessary to limit or avoid the use of oil for several months until health improves.

BEANS

Beans and their products, including tofu, tempeh, natto, and others, comprise about 5 to 10 percent of the standard macrobiotic diet. Any of the following varieties may be selected:

Regular Use

Azuki beans
Bean products
Black soybeans
Chickpeas (Garbanzo beans)
Dried tofu (soybean curd that has been naturally dried)
Fresh tofu
Lentils (green)
Natto (fermented soybeans)
Tempeh (fermented soybeans or combination of soybeans and grains)

Occasional Use

Black-eyed peas
Black turtle beans
Great northern beans
Kidney beans
Mung beans
Navy beans
Pinto beans
Soybeans
Split peas
Whole dried peas

Beans and bean products are more easily digested when cooked with a small volume of seasonings such as sea salt, miso, or kombu sea vegetable. They may also be prepared with vegetables, chestnuts, dried apples, or raisins, and occasionally sweetened with grain sweeteners like barley malt and rice honey. Serve them in soups and side dishes, or with grains or sea vegetables.

Cancer-Inhibiting Properties

Epidemiological studies indicate that regular consumption of pulses (the edible seeds of certain pod-bearing plants), such as lentils, reduces risk of cancer. In addition, soybeans, a major source of protein in the macrobiotic diet, have been singled out as especially effective in reducing tumors. As with whole grains, protease inhibitors are the active ingredients in soybeans. Laboratory tests show that adding soybeans and certain other beans and seeds containing these inhibitors to the diet prevents the development of breast, stomach, colon, liver, and skin tumors. Whole soybeans and soy products, including miso, tamari soy sauce, tofu, tempeh, and natto, are staples of the macrobiotic diet.

General Guidelines

Beans from the "Regular Use" column can be eaten daily, as can tofu, dried tofu, tempeh, and other bean products. Those in the "Occasional Use" column can be eaten two or three times per month, on average. Beans are more digestible when cooked with kombu sea vegetable.

SEA VEGETABLES

Sea vegetables provide essential minerals and may be used daily in cooking. Arame and hijiki make wonderful side dishes and can be included several times per week. Wakame and kombu can be used daily in miso and other soups, in vegetable and bean dishes, or in making condiments. Toasted nori is a good source of iron and is also recommended for daily or regular use. Agar-agar can be used from time to time in making a natural jelled dessert known as kanten. Below is a list of sea vegetables used in macrobiotic cooking:

Regular Use (daily)

Kombu	Wakame
Toasted nori	

Regular use (several times per week)

Arame   Hijiki

Optional Use

Agar-agar   Sea palm
Dulse   Other traditionally
Irish moss   used sea
Mekabu   vegetables

Cancer-Inhibiting Properties

Medical studies and case reports indicate that sea vegetables can be effective in eliminating tumors. In 1974, in the *Japanese Journal of Experimental Medicine*, scientists stated that several varieties of kombu (a common sea vegetable eaten in Asia and in macrobiotic diets) were effective in the treatment of tumors. In three of four samples tested in the lab, inhibition rates in mice with implanted cancerous tumors ranged from 89 to 95 percent. The researchers reported, "The tumor underwent complete regression in more than half of the mice of each treated group." Similiar experiments, in which mice with leukemia were treated with sea vegetables, showed promising results. A 1986 screening of sea vegetables for antitumor activity found that nine out of the eleven varieties studied inhibited tumors in animals.

In 1984, medical researcher Dr. Jane Teas and associates at the Harvard School of Public Health reported that a diet containing 5 percent kombu significantly delayed the inducement of breast cancer in experimental animals. Extrapolating these results to human subjects, the investigators concluded, "Seaweed may be an important factor in explaining the low rates of certain types of cancers in Japan." Japanese women, whose diet normally includes about 5 percent sea vegetables, have an incidence of breast cancer that is from three to nine times lower than the rate among American women, whose diet does not normally include sea vegetables. Dr. Teas and researchers in Japan believe that a chemical called fucoidan

The Anti-Radiation Effects of Sea Vegetables

Plants from the sea may protect against radioactivity. Medical doctors in Nagasaki who, after the atomic bombing in 1945, helped save their patients on a traditional diet of brown rice, miso soup, and sea vegetables attested to this. In addition, scientists at McGill University in Canada reported in the 1960s and 1970s that common edible sea vegetables contained a substance that selectively combined with radioactive strontium and helped eliminate it naturally from the body. The substance, sodium alginate, was prepared from kombu, kelp, and other brown sea vegetables found in Atlantic and Pacific coastal waters. "The evaluation of biological activity of different marine algae is important because of their practical significance in preventing absorption of radioactive products of atomic fission as well as in the use of possible natural decontaminators," the researchers concluded in an article in the *Canadian Medical Association Journal.*

may be the most potent among the various anticancer agents contained in sea vegetables.

Studies of wakame, commonly used in miso soup and in other macrobiotic dishes, have also revealed antitumor activity. Scientists at the University of Hawaii discovered that when injected into mice, dried wakame prevented and reversed lung cancer.

General Guidelines

A small volume of sea vegetables can be eaten daily. One-half to one sheet of toasted nori can be eaten in soups, in homemade sushi or rice balls, or as a garnish for other dishes. Kombu and wakame can be used daily in miso and other soups and in preparing beans and other dishes. Side dishes made from arame or hijiki can be prepared two or three times per week. The sea vegetables in the "Optional Use" category can also be included from time to time.

WHITE-MEAT FISH

Low-fat, white-meat fish can be eaten on occasion to supplement the foods already listed. Amounts eaten can vary, depending upon your needs and desires, but generally, several times per week is sufficient. White-meat varieties that are lowest in fat and most easily digested are recommended for regular use.

Ocean Varieties

Cod	Scrod
Flounder	Shad
Haddock	Smelt
Halibut	Sole
Herring	Other varieties
Ocean trout	of white-meat
Perch	ocean fish

Freshwater Varieties

Bass	Trout
Carp	Whitefish
Catfish	Other varieties of white-
Pike	meat, freshwater fish

Garnishes are especially important in balancing fish and seafood. Recommended garnishes for persons in good health include: chopped scallions or parsley, grated raw daikon, ginger, radish, or horseradish, green mustard paste (wasabi), raw salad, and shredded daikon.

General Guidelines

Overconsumption of fat and protein from animal sources is a leading contributor to cancer. Therefore, it is generally advisable to limit the intake of low-fat, white-meat fish to once a week until the condition improves. Among the recommended garnishes for fish, a tablespoonful or two of grated raw daikon radish is preferred. Steamed or boiled fish (as in fish soup) is preferable to broiled, baked, or grilled fish. Deep-fried fish is best avoided. In certain cases, for example, following chemotherapy or if a person is experiencing weight loss due to illness, the recommended frequency of white-meat fish can be increased.

FRUIT

In most cases, fruit can be enjoyed three or four times per week. Locally grown or temperate climate fruits are preferable, while tropical fruits are not recommended for regular use by people in temperate regions. Below are varieties for consumption in temperate climates:

Regular Use

Apples	Peaches
Apricots	Plums
Blackberries	Raisins
Cantaloupe	Raspberries
Grapes	Strawberries
Honeydew melon	Tangerines
Lemons	Watermelon
Mulberries	Wild berries
Persimmon	

To Avoid in a Temperate Climate

Banana	Pineapple
Dates	Other tropical or
Figs	semitropical fruits

General Guidelines

In order to recover health, the intake of simple sugars, including those in fruit, is best kept to a minimum. In general, until good health is reestablished, it is best to eat fruit only to satisfy cravings. "The less the better" is a good maxim to observe until health is restored. When fruit is craved, a small serving of northern fruit cooked with a pinch of sea salt can be eaten.

Prayer, Faith, and Macrobiotics

My life embarked on a new path on July 1st, 1987, when the urologist, during a very painful examination, declared that he would have to take a biopsy at the hospital because my urethra contained a tumor he was sure was malignant. He advised me to go home and talk with my family, but to enter Baylor Hospital the following Monday at 6 A.M.

My first reaction was disbelief, since I seemed so healthy, except for this nagging pressure on my bladder, and because no one in my entire family had ever had cancer. I thought the doctor was probably mistaken! My husband and I were both in shock! However, I soon felt a deep spiritual calm and assurance that God was in control and that He would direct our path.

During the next few days, we talked and prayed with my five grown children and then with my husband's three, plus our sisters and brothers and their families. Comfort and support from close friends and family help so much when you are devastated.

On July 3rd, my husband and I had lunch at our favorite health food store, as we had so many times before. This time, from an open book rack, the book *The Cancer Prevention Diet* seemed to be leaping out to me. I took it and flipped through it, thinking that I would buy it in order to compare what the author had to say with our "healthy" diet of almost all raw foods. I also wanted to hear what the author had to say about cancer prevention. We had never heard of Michio Kushi or macrobiotics before.

On Monday morning, July 6, the biopsy proved the doctor to be correct. The diagnosis was a Stage III carcinoma of the urethra that had spread to the bladder. The doctor explained that this was a very rare cancer and extremely lethal. He felt it was most important to proceed quickly with all that was medically possible for the condition.

First, he set me up with the head radiologist, who decided that a radium implant—the maximum for seven days—would be done on July 8. During my stay at Baylor Hospital, everyone was caring and efficient, but I was so sick with intense pain and nausea. Pain medication provided only temporary relief.

On July 17th, my radiologist removed the implants and inserted a new catheter that remained in place for the next several weeks. After I left the hospital, the doctor checked me weekly and showed concern when, after six weeks, my strength had not returned. He and my urologist started planning and pressing me to have radical surgery by the following month.

I explained to the doctors that I was following a wonderful macrobiotic diet, but their reaction was that I was "too intelligent to believe that a diet or food had anything to do with cancer remission." Meanwhile, my husband found a macrobiotic center in Dallas and took cooking classes and bought supplies and books describing macrobiotic cancer recoveries. Thankfully, my husband, J.R., had always liked to cook and had been something of a "health nut." So we embarked together on this new way of cooking, eating, and learning.

So It was only natural that I desired to go to Boston to meet with Michio Kushi. We called the Kushi Foundation and were able to meet with him on August 23. I was still quite weak and the united message from most of my famliy and friends was to "put myself in the doctors' hands, since they know best."

During our meeting, Mr. Kushi was cautiously optimistic. He felt that I would improve if I followed the macrobiotic recommendations, and he suggested modifications in my diet along with home-care preparations. He recommended walking for a half-hour each day, and suggested that I sing a happy song every day to keep my spirits up. He also emphasized chewing each mouthful at least fifty times.

Upon returning to Dallas, we followed Mr. Kushi's suggestions to the letter. We decided on our own to delay the surgery and see how things went. Gradually, my health and strength returned, and each visit to the doctor confirmed that the tumor was shrinking! In October, my doctor presented my case before the Dallas Board of Urologists. He felt that additional medical opinions would convince me of the urgency and necessity of radical surgery. I told him I appreciated his concern.

Shortly afterward, he called to report that all the doctors were of the opinion that surgery was critical to save my life, and that it must take place before December or else it would be too late. The reason I was so reluctant to have radical surgery was that it involved approximately sixteen hours of surgery, and seemingly one-fourth of my body would be cut out. Even with all this, my chances of surviving five years or longer were slim, and I was as concerned with the quality of life as I was with the quantity of years.

Early in November, we again went to see Mr. Kushi. He was delighted with my progress and was very optimistic about the chances for recovery. Again, we went home and continued very strictly on our healing diet. We prayed every step of the way, and I also walked two miles daily and laughed and sang. I did not call the doctor again, for he advised me not to until I had agreed to have surgery.

By the following June (1988), after returning home from

Florida, I went to see the doctor. He was glad to see me and surprised to see how well and radiant I was. After conducting a cystoscopy, CAT scans, x-rays, and blood work, he exclaimed that he was shocked and amazed that all the tests were clear—for now! He also said that my case would go into medical books, because no one with this condition had ever lived this long without radical surgery following the radium implant. I asked if he were just a little curious about what I had been doing during this time, but he just smiled and said, "Barbara, your body reacted extremely well to the radium implant, and I know that you have great faith, but for sure, it is not that health diet you are on."

Upon leaving the doctor's office, J.R. and I were so excited that we jumped for joy and praised the Lord! There was rejoicing everywhere and with everyone. At a meeting of our macrobiotic group, everyone stood up and applauded and hugged us. The members of our church, as well as our family and friends who had prayed so faithfully for my healing, all rejoiced and shed many tears of thankfulness with us.

Since 1988, we have attended the annual Macrobiotic Summer Conference held in the Berkshire Mountains of Massachusetts. I have told my story in front of a large audience several times. A number of people with cancer who were attending the Conference told me that my story encouraged and inspired them. These experiences have been overwhelming, and since that time, telling my story to encourage others has become my ministry. In 1988, we started a cancer support group, the Lifeline, in order to help others. We started with only four people, and then it quickly grew to ten, and then twenty-five, and beyond!

In April 1990, I told my story on a television show in Atlanta. Before going to Atlanta, I went to the doctor for an exam. He completed a cystoscopy and was amazed that the walls of my bladder were soft and pliable rather than rigid because of scar tissue. He said he saw no need for any further tests because it was clear that I had recovered. He stated that I was a "medical miracle."

In conclusion, the last three years have been some of the best years of my life. I feel deepest gratitude toward everyone and everything that contributed to my recovery: Michio Kushi, my expert doctors, the nutritionally balanced macrobiotic diet, physical exercise, and most importantly, the prayers and faith of my family and friends.

If fresh fruit is craved during the summer, a small volume can be eaten with a pinch of sea salt sprinkled on it. The intake of raw fruit is best kept to a minimum.

PICKLES

Pickles can be eaten frequently as a supplement to main dishes. They stimulate appetite and help digestion. Some varieties—such as pickled daikon, or takuan—can be bought prepackaged in natural food stores. Others—such as quick pickles—can be prepared at home.

Regular Use

Amazake pickles	Rice bran pickles
Brine pickles	Sauerkraut
Miso pickles	Takuan pickles
Pressed pickles	Tamari soy sauce pickles

Avoid (for Optimal Health)

Dill pickles	Spiced pickles
Garlic pickles	Vinegar pickles
Herb pickles	

General Guidelines

One tablespoonful of naturally processed, non-spicy pickles can be eaten daily. If pickles have a strong salty flavor, rinse them quickly under cold water before eating.

SEEDS AND NUTS

Seeds and nuts can be eaten from time to time as snacks and garnishes. They can be roasted with or without sea salt, sweetened with barley or rice malt, or seasoned with tamari soy sauce. Seeds and nuts can be ground into butter, shaved and served as a topping or garnish, or used as an ingredient in various dishes, including dessert. Below are varieties that can be used:

Regular Use

Almonds	Pecans
Black and white	Pine nuts
sesame seeds	Pumpkin seeds
Chestnuts	Small Spanish nuts
Filberts	Squash seeds
Peanuts	Sunflower seeds
	Walnuts

Infrequent Use

Brazil nuts	Macadamia nuts
Cashews	Others

General Guidelines

With the exception of chestnuts, nuts are high in oils and fats. Therefore, it is better to minimize or avoid eating them until health is restored. Chestnuts, however, can be eaten from time to time for a naturally sweet taste. Up to a cup and a half of lightly roasted, unsalted seeds can be eaten per week. Sunflower seeds are best eaten only during the summer months and not until health is restored.

SNACKS

A variety of natural snacks may be enjoyed from time to time, including those made from whole grains, like cookies, bread, puffed cereals, mochi (cakes made of pounded sweet brown rice), rice cakes, rice balls, and homemade sushi. Lightly roasted nuts and seeds may also be eaten as snacks. The following natural snacks are fine for regular use:

Leftovers	Rice balls
Mochi	Rice cakes
Noodles	Seeds
Popcorn (homemade	Sushi (made at home
and unbuttered)	without sugar, seasoning,
Puffed whole cereal	or MSG)
grains	Steamed sourdough bread

The Balance
of Natural Flavors

The naturally sweet taste of whole grains, beans, vegetables such as carrots, squash, and cabbage, sea vegetables, and other whole foods is the most important of natural flavors. Natural sweetness is derived from complex carbohydrates, which make up our primary nutritional requirement, and is the hub around which the other tastes revolve. It is usually the predominant flavor at each meal, while other flavors can be used for variety or to highlight and bring forth the natural sweetness of your dishes. In the table below, we present the most common sources for the five primary tastes.

Flavor	Primary Sources
Naturally sweet	Whole grains, beans, naturally sweet vegetables (e.g., cabbage, squash, carrots, onions)
Sour	Naturally fermented foods (e.g., umeboshi plum, brown rice and umeboshi vinegar, pickled vegetables, sauerkraut)
Bitter	Green leafy vegetables (e.g., mustard greens, dandelion greens, watercress), burdock, roasted condiments
Spicy	Raw chopped scallions, ginger, grated raw daikon
Salty	Sea salt, including condiments and seasonings such as miso, tamari soy sauce, gomashio, umeboshi plum, tekka, and others processed with sea salt

If the supplemental tastes (sour, bitter, spicy, and salty) are used too strongly—by adding too much miso, tamari, or sea salt to foods, for example, or by using too many salty condiments—the patient may begin to crave the artifically sweet taste of refined and other simple sugars. This craving will make it more difficult for the patient to comfortably stay within the guidelines of macrobiotics. For maximum health and enjoyment, therefore, try to emphasize the gentle, natural sweetness of whole natural foods at every meal and use the other flavors in moderation.

General Guidelines

Snacks that have a drying or tightening effect on the body, such as popcorn, puffed cereals, or rice cakes, are best eaten in moderation. Other snacks can be enjoyed as desired. However, avoid snacking for $2^1/2$ to 3 hours before sleeping.

CONDIMENTS

A variety of condiments may be used, some daily and others occasionally. Small amounts can be sprinkled on foods to adjust taste and nutritional value, and to stimulate appetite. They can be used on grains, soups, vegetables, beans, and sometimes desserts. The most frequently used varieties include:

Regular Use

Gomashio (roasted sesame seeds and sea salt)

Tekka (a special condiment made with soybean miso, sesame oil, burdock, lotus root, carrots, and ginger)

Green nori flakes

Sea vegetable powders (with or without roasted sesame seeds)

Umeboshi (salty, pickled plums)

Occasional Use

Cooked miso with scallions or onions

Cooked nori condiment

Roasted and chopped shiso (pickled beefsteak plant) leaves

Roasted sesame seeds

Shio kombu (kombu cooked with tamari and water)

Umeboshi or brown rice vinegar

General Guidelines

"Regular Use" condiments can be kept on the table and added to whole grain and other dishes as desired. Gomashio (sesame salt) and roasted sea vegetable powders can be sprinkled on dishes as you would salt and pepper. About one teaspoonful of these sprinkled condiments can be used daily. Tekka is a stronger condiment and is best used moderately, about a teaspoonful or so per week, on average. Two or three umeboshi plums can be eaten per week along with grains or other dishes. "Occasional Use" condiments can be used about two or three times per week if desired for variety. Condiments that include sea salt are best used in moderation.

SEASONINGS

It is better to avoid strong spicy seasonings such as curry, hot pepper, and others, and to use those which are naturally processed from vegetable products or natural sea salt, and which have been used as a part of traditional diets. A list of seasonings recommended in the standard macrobiotic diet is presented below:

Regular Use

Miso (fermented soybean and grain paste, i.e., rice, barley, soybean, sesame, and other misos)

Soy sauce
Tamari soy sauce (fermented soybean and grain sauce)
Unrefined sea salt

Occasional Use

Brown rice and umeboshi vinegar
Garlic
Grated daikon, radish, and ginger
Lemon

Mirin (fermented sweet brown rice liquid)
Sesame and corn oil
Umeboshi plum and paste
Other traditional natural seasonings

Avoid (for Optimal Health)

Commercial seasonings
Irradiated spices and herbs

Stimulant and aromatic spices and herbs

General Guidelines

In general, use seasonings in moderation. Dishes should have a mild, not salty, flavor. A moderate amount of "Regular Use" seasonings can be used daily in cooking; those in the "Occasional Use" column can be used several times per week for variety. Mirin, which contains a small amount of alcohol, is best avoided temporarily by those seeking to improve their health. Raw garlic is best avoided.

SWEETS

The naturally sweet flavor of cooked vegetables can be featured daily for optimal health. Include one or several of the vegetables listed below:

Cabbage	Pumpkin
Carrots	Squash
Daikon	Sweet vegetable
Onions	drink
Parsnips	or jam

In addition, a small amount of concentrated sweeteners made from whole cereal grains may be included when desired. Dried chestnuts, which also impart a sweet flavor, may also be included on occasion, along with occasional apple juice or cider. Additional natural sweeteners include:

Amazake	Chestnuts (cooked)
Barley malt	Hot apple cider
Brown rice syrup	Hot apple juice

General Guidelines

The best quality sweets are those derived from the complex carbohydrates in whole grains and naturally sweet vegetables, and foods such as chestnuts. Naturally sweet vegetables can be included in various dishes on a daily basis. In addition, sweet vegetable drink (see inset page 127) can also be used daily or often to relieve the craving for sweets. A small amount of concentrated sweeteners, including grain syrups, amazake, and apple juice, can be used on occasion to relieve the craving for sweets.

BEVERAGES

A variety of beverages may be consumed daily or occasionally. Amounts can vary according to weather conditions and each person's needs. The beverages listed below can be used to comfortably satisfy the desire for liquid.

Regular Use

Bancha stem tea
Bancha twig tea
 (kukicha)
High-quality natural
 well water

Natural spring
 water (suitable for
 daily use)
Roasted brown rice
 or barley tea

Occasional Use

Dandelion tea
Freshly squeezed
 carrot juice
 (if desired,
 about two cups
 per week)

Grain coffee (100 percent
 roasted cereal grains)
Kombu tea
Mu tea
Sweet vegetable broth
Umeboshi tea

Infrequent Use

Beer (natural quality)
Green leaf tea
Green magma (barley
 green juice)
Northern climate
 fruit juice

Sake (fermented rice
 wine, without chemicals
 or sugar)
Soymilk
Vegetable juice
Wine (natural quality)

Avoid (for Optimal Health)

Aromatic herbal teas	Hard liquor
Chemically colored tea	Mineral water and all bubbling waters
Chemically processed beverages	Stimulant beverages
Coffee	Sugared drinks
Cold or iced drinks	Tap water
Distilled water	Tropical fruit juices

General Guidelines

Beverages in the "Regular Use" column can be enjoyed on a daily basis, while those in the "Occasional Use" column can be enjoyed two or three times per week. Those suggested for infrequent use are best avoided until health becomes normal.

PROPER COOKING

Macrobiotic cooking is quick and simple once a few basic techniques — how to use a pressure cooker, wash and cut vegetables, and how to plan menus to ensure adequate taste and variety — are mastered. Before you learn the basics, however, it is easy to make mistakes. This is especially true when getting started, since many of the foods and cooking methods are often new and unfamiliar. However, you will develop proficiency in this skill — as in any other — once you become familiar with the ingredients and methods used in macrobiotic cooking.

Recipes and cookbooks are, of course, helpful, but the best way to learn about macrobiotic cooking is to attend classes where you can actually see the foods prepared and can taste them. Most introductory macrobiotic cooking classes are presented in a series of six to eight sessions, and will show you how to do important things like wash and soak foods, cut vegetables, purée miso for soup, and combine ingredients in complete meals. Advice on menu planning, setting up your

Cookbooks Can Help

There are a number of books that may prove helpful in learning about the principles and practices of macrobiotics. For home study, the following cookbooks are especially recommended:

☐ *Aveline Kushi's Complete Guide to Macrobiotic Cooking*, by Aveline Kushi with Alex Jack, Warner Books, 1985.

☐ *Aveline Kushi's Introducing Macrobiotic Cooking*, by Aveline Kushi with Wendy Esko, Japan Publications, 1987.

☐ *Aveline Kushi's Wonderful World of Salads*, by Aveline Kushi and Wendy Esko, Japan Publications, 1989.

☐ *The Changing Seasons Macrobiotic Cookbook*, by Aveline Kushi and Wendy Esko, Avery Publishing Group, 1985.

☐ *The Good Morning Macrobiotic Breakfast Book*, by Aveline Kushi and Wendy Esko, Avery Publishing Group, 1991.

☐ *The Macrobiotic Cancer Prevention Cookbook*, by Aveline Kushi with Wendy Esko, Avery Publishing Group, 1988.

☐ *Macrobiotic Cooking for Everyone*, by Edward and Wendy Esko, Japan Publications, 1980.

☐ *The New Pasta Cuisine: Low-Fat Noodle and Pasta Dishes From Around the World*, by Aveline Kushi and Wendy Esko, Japan Publications, 1991.

☐ *The Quick and Natural Macrobiotic Cookbook*, by Aveline Kushi and Wendy Esko, Contemporary Books, 1989.

kitchen, and shopping for high-quality foods is usually provided as well.

Weekly dinners, which many macrobiotic centers sponsor, are also helpful, as they offer you the chance to see and taste a balanced meal and to talk to other people about macrobiotics in a relaxed and supportive setting. Some programs, such as the Macrobiotic Residential Seminar presented by the Kushi Institute in the Berkshires, offer a combination of meals and hands-on cooking training. Programs that offer hands-on guidance are the best for learning to cook properly.

7

Recovery and Beyond

When we come to analyze the conception of disease in society or in the individual, it evidently means *loss of unity*. Health, therefore, should mean unity, and it is curious that the history of the word entirely corroborates this idea. The words health, whole, holy are from the same stock; and they indicate that far back in the past those who created this group of words had a conception of health very different from ours.

Edward Carpenter
Civilization: Its Cause and Cure

The many exceptional cancer patients I have met over the years all share a variety of common factors that aided them in recovery. In this, our concluding chapter, we look at the main features shared by these exceptional patients, and discuss the new dimensions of health that come from living in harmony with nature.

UNDERSTANDING AND SENSITIVITY

Most exceptional cancer patients are well-informed about their illness and the options available to them. They adopt macrobiotics freely and wholeheartedly after reviewing the evidence and arriving at their own conclusions. Backed by their own knowledge and awareness, they become active participants in creating health.

Changing previous dietary and lifestyle habits requires patience, sensitivity, and understanding. It is important for someone with a serious illness to practice the macrobiotic guidelines accurately. This requires putting forth effort to study and master the principles of macrobiotics, along with basic cooking, in order to understand why food is important and how it affects our health. The patient needs to be cautious — in the sense of avoiding unbalanced foods that impede recovery — but not rigid or narrow. Eating the full range of foods within the guidelines of macrobiotics helps maintain the necessary flexibility, as does using a wide range of cooking methods.

Creating varied and balanced meals is, of course, an immediate priority for the sick person and his family. It is important for the patient to have enough variety to maintain interest and enthusiasm, and to satisfy nutritional requirements. Food should be enjoyable, and by focusing on the addition and discovery of new foods, rather than on the omission of old ones, the practice of macrobiotics becomes an exciting adventure and continuous learning process.

SPIRITUAL AWARENESS

Exceptional cancer patients are genuinely grateful for their illness and what it has to teach them. They do not complain and blame others, but look within themselves for the source of their troubles. They realize the shortcomings of their past way of eating and living and are happy to make a fresh start and change. Such people often have a deep faith in something larger than themselves, such as God, nature, or the universe, and they experience the coming of macrobiotics into their lives as an expression of that faith. As their health improves, they grow closer to their original religious heritage, and their appreciation of other spiritual traditions deepens. After healing themselves, such people often go on to help many others.

Looking back on their illness, they often say that cancer was one of the best things that ever happened to them because of the changes it brought in their understanding of life.

Difficulty and suffering can also strengthen our spiritual capacities. People who have experienced the full range of pain and fear and who truly want to be free from suffering readily embrace the diet. They have tried many different symptomatic approaches and have been disappointed. They are now ready to give up their defensive way of life, their stubbornness, and their rigidity to find freedom and regain their health. They have developed the ability to self-reflect and have embarked on a personal search for health and truth. When they discover the unifying principle of yin and yang, they learn how to transmute sickness into health and sorrow into joy.

WILL AND DETERMINATION

People who have cancer and still retain their cheerfulness, humor, and will to live also have a high likelihood of success. These people usually have very strong native constitutions that they inherited from parents and ancestors who ate grains and vegetables as a major portion of their diet. This shows up in such features as a large head, firm bone structure (especially in men), steady well-focused eyes, proportionately large hands, and large ears that lie flat against the side of the head and have long, detached lobes. Even though such persons spoiled their health in later life, they have reservoirs of strength from their embryological development and early childhood. They also have a foundation of common sense and appreciation, which they have lately forgotten. They only need to be reminded.

If a person with a strong will feels powerless in the face of disease, he or she may react with anger and hostility. Studies have shown that some long-term survivors of breast cancer, for example, evidence a greater degree of "fighting spirit," and have higher scores for hostility and other negative feelings than short-term survivors. Along with having more negative attitudes toward their cancer, they often have a poorer attitude toward their doctors. These strong emotions, as in all of

A New Education

"John, do you think she'll make it."

"No, because she has handed this over to you. She is letting you take care of it."

This conversation occurred one morning in February 1987 when my husband, David, and our host, John Carter, were driving me to a macrobiotic seminar in Brookline, Massachusetts. I was supposed to be asleep in the back seat. David was asking John what my chances were of recovering from a fast-growing brain tumor.

David answered John by saying, "I don't understand that. She has always been an independent person, in fact, too independent."

I realized right then that I had to take over! No more would the doctors or David direct my life; no more would I feel like a bump on a log when David and the doctors discussed *my* case. I would take charge.

In August of 1986, everything was wonderful. I had just turned thirty-seven and was thoroughly enjoying life. I loved everything about it and was having a wonderful time. And then the bottom fell out.

After a grand mal seizure that sent me sprawling onto an asphalt tennis court, many, many tests in two hospitals, and two surgeries, I was diagnosed as having a grade 3 anaplastic astrocytoma. This is a fast-growing inoperative brain tumor. At that time it was about the size of a small grapefruit.

Tumor . . . Tumor . . . the name kept jumping out at me like a 3-D movie, visible—but untouchable. Through all of the discussions of the abnormality, tumor or cancer had never been a possibility in my mind. The reality hit home when I was asked to visit a "tumor center" for discussion of possible treatments for *my* brain tumor—*my* cancer.

To say that the discovery that I had cancer was an earthshaking experience is an understatement. I think the impact of the diagnosis caused me, one night soon after, to experience a series of physical jolts: nausea, vomiting, and numbness in my right leg. The emotional trauma was something that I was not accustomed to.

I've always been a contented, happy person, able to see the bright side of things, even while "bitching." I could find contentment sitting on a rock at Smith Lake or dancing in my husband's arms in romantic places like Bermuda. I had always enjoyed life, living by my own decisions—until now.

The doctors said it was bad . . . would never go away—chemotherapy could hopefully only slow its growth—was close to motor area . . . would lose motor control . . . wheelchair in future . . . six to eighteen months to live . . . downhill all the way. It was worse than a Freddie Kruger nightmare. I couldn't wake up.

It did not belong there. I wanted *it* gone.

When my aunt from New Orleans suggested macrobiotics, I had no idea what she was talking about and the idea that food could make a malignancy go away was absurd. But when you have no alternative and a strong desire to live, you do whatever you can.

So, I read *Recalled By Life* by Anthony Sattilaro, as my aunt suggested, and later read *Recovery* by Elaine Nussbaum. Elaine was a housewife like me but in much worse shape. I reasoned that if she could recover, I could, too. It did not matter that I lived in a small town in northeast Mississippi and knew no one who had even heard of macrobiotics at that time.

Before jumping right in, though, I decided I would give the American Cancer Society hotline a final check to see if there were anything else I could do. At this point I had had six-thousand RADs and two treatments of chemo (PCNU). At least five more treatments were scheduled.

The hotline volunteer answered, "Nothing. Good luck." The line went dead.

Through clenched teeth my reply was, "We'll see about that!"

Three days later, January 17, 1987, I was on my way to the Macrobiotic Learning Center in Brookline, Massachusetts. This beginner course was given in a home that to me, a Mississippi native, seemed damp and chilly. I had trouble understanding the various foreign teachers and the fast-talking Yankee instructors, and, of course, they couldn't understand my Southern accent. The ingredients for the meals could have come from another planet, and I had trouble eating and enjoying the food.

At that time I was on many antiseizure pills and my thinking was clouded, to say the least. Luckily, I had taken my camcorder and taped everything, because trying to absorb everything sent me to bed with a headache each night.

In short, this was not a pleasant experience, but I would not go back to Mississippi and say that. This was my chance to live and I was going to take it.

Looking back now, I am able to realize how much I absorbed, and I credit much of my success to that program. I learned not only the proper way to cook, but also exercises, massage, home remedies, and the power of positive thinking.

So back to Columbus, Mississippi, I went, ready to get under way with my new macrobiotic life. After unpacking all the videos I'd made and the books and tapes I'd purchased, I was ready to begin.

I was quick to learn that cooking alone was quite different from having an ever-ready teacher plus six other students in the kitchen. I started my first solo macro meal at 3 P.M. I finished a little after 8 P.M., at which time I was too exhausted to eat!

Another turning point came when I returned to Boston in February to see Michio Kushi. It was then that I overheard the conversation mentioned at the start of this article.

Taking charge meant that I was going to stop taking chemotherapy and that I was going to get off the nine antiseizure pills and tachycardia medicine I was supposed to take for the rest of my life.

I had to tell the neuro-oncologist and my husband, David, about my decision to discontinue the chemo. The antiseizure medication had to be gradually decreased and I didn't want to tell them until I had been off it and the tachycardia pills for a month. This took a year and when I told them what I had done, they had a fit. But all's been well.

Well—almost all: That first winter, my mind was so drugged that I couldn't get from the cookbook to the stove without forgetting what to do. I kept feeling worse and worse and colder and colder. But I said I'd try it for six months, and six months it was going to be.

From somewhere came the idea of hiring a macrobiotic cook. After numerous calls to John Carter and reference checks, Dawn Gilmour arrived from Boston, and some of the food actually started tasting good!

Dawn gave me some concoctions I'd read about but never tried. One, a simple drink made with heated apple juice and diluted kuzu, had a wonderful calming effect.

Dawn was a normal person with hopes, dreams, and fears like the rest of us, which meant I could identify with her and, at the same time, learn from her.

The only regret I have is that during the week Dawn was with me, I would get terribly tired during meal preparation and would end up taking a nap. I don't know if this was a defense mechanism or what, but thank the Lord for Mamie.

Mamie was a wonderful woman who I'm sure was sent to me from God. In fact before she came to work for us, I was in a "dither" getting ready for Dawn's arrival and, as always, was running out of time and energy. As I stood in our breakfast room I said, "Lord, what am I going to do?"

Mamie rang the doorbell to introduce herself to me. (I had

hired her a few days earlier, sight unseen.) She had been on the way to town and had just decided to stop. I promptly hugged her and started crying. She then came into the house in her "town clothes" and helped me prepare for Dawn.

Of course, Mamie was there for Dawn's teaching and absorbed it all. Mamie had a superb memory and was a wonderful cook.

She also was like a mother to me; she would make me sit down and plan the day's menu, making sure I was eating all I was supposed to and getting the rest I needed. I truly do not know what I would have done without her guidance and persistence.

Macrobiotics was a challenge for me. Slowly, through training by the experts and experimenting on my own, I learned that I could make delicious meals that would enable me to enjoy the food while my body was healing itself.

I stopped the chemotherapy after the third treatment and began a full-time holistic regime to heal my body and soul.

A verse from Ephesians in the Bible became my motto: "Now unto Him that is able to do exceedingly abundantly above all that we ask or think, according to the power that worketh in us." God had given me the power to take charge of my life again and to make myself well.

Besides prayer and macrobiotics, I used imaging. I also used a video tape and a subliminal cassette that both constantly told me the tumor was decreasing. In my bedroom, I kept a drawing of the tumor that showed it decreasing in size—from the size of a grapefruit to a golfball to a pinhead to nothing! Amazingly, each test showed the size of the malignancy had diminished just as I had drawn.

The CAT scan made in April of 1987, four months after I had started macrobiotics, showed no evidence of cancer! And no scans have since then, either.

One night two years ago, my nine-year-old son, Parker, asked, "Mom, do you think you'll ever get cancer again?"

My immediate reply was, "No." After a bit I came back into his bedroom and added, "But, Parker, don't worry, honey, because if I do, I know what to do."

He smiled and said, "We'll fight like before."

It's wonderful to have that assurance. In a way the feeling can be compared to seeing a rainbow after a storm and remembering God's promise.

My healing process was not just luck. It was my strong faith in God, the many prayers sent for me and by me, my determination, a positive outlook, imaging, video and subliminal tapes, and the accurate practice of the macrobiotic diet.

It was also the love and support of my husband, children, family, and of friends who became so close they felt like sisters. It was realizing that I, not anyone else, was responsible for my health. No one thing can control cancer: not just diet, not just radiation, not just chemotherapy. The body heals itself with God's help. I used everything else as tools.

Through all these things, I have regained my physical, mental, and spiritual health.

I am alive with the chance to work, play, and love, and I want to share my experience with others to spare them the anguish I went through and to offer an alternative to degenerative disease.

Source: "Healing a Terminal Brain Tumor," *One Peaceful World*, Autumn/Winter, 1990; correspondence with Mona Sanders, Columbus, Mississippi, August 30, 1990.

---

us, are a vehicle for discharging excess. Crying, for example, is a way of eliminating toxic substances from the body. Emotional tears contain more protein than those caused by irritants such as dust. By expressing their emotions rather than holding them in, the long-term survivors are able to discharge some of the excess that would have accelerated the growth of their cancers. In addition, as they begin to understand the underlying causes of their illness, rather than being powerless they are empowered, and can channel their "fighting spirit" in a constructive direction by taking positive action to restore their health.

LOVE AND CARE OF FAMILY AND FRIENDS

With the close cooperation and support of the patient's immediate family, the possibility of recovery is greatly enhanced. The patient's family should clearly understand the situation and begin to eat in a similar manner, while extending love and support to the patient in every possible way.

It is well known that persons with disrupted or weakened social and family ties have an increased susceptibility to disease. This phenomenon is described by Robert Ornstein, Ph.D., and David Sobel, M.D., in *The Healing Brain*:

> People who are single, separated, divorced, or widowed are two or three times more likely to die than their married peers. They also wind up in the hospital for mental disorders five to ten times as frequently. Whether we look at heart disease, cancer, depression, tuberculosis, arthritis, or problems during pregnancy, the occurance of disease is higher in those with weakened social connectedness.

A warm, loving, and supportive family provides an environment that encourages health and recovery.

When caring for others we need to keep in mind that the object of healing is to improve our own health and understanding, as well as the patient's. Dealing with serious illness can be draining. However, at some level we are receiving as much energy as we give out. Helping someone with cancer challenges our own understanding of the universe as well as our physical stamina, mental clarity, and emotional strength.

The macrobiotic approach provides a clear and hopeful direction. However, it is usually up to the immediate family members to help the patient implement that direction, make day-to-day decisions about what to cook, how to apply home care, and how to handle whatever problems or crises may come up. Family members or friends who take care of the person with cancer also need to constantly self-reflect and consider whether their advice is sound. As we develop as healers and teachers, we will face many difficulties and frustrations. However, as our own way of eating improves and our intuition develops, we will be able to help more and more people.

NEW DIMENSIONS OF HEALTH

Recovering from illness is only the first step in the ongoing process of achieving genuine health. For many of us in the modern world, health is defined in the negative sense as the absence of illness. Positive aspects—including the establishment

of harmony in mind, body, and spirit and the joyful and creative adaptation to the environment are often missing from the
modern definition. As the 19th-century English writer Edward
Carpenter pointed out in *Civilization: Its Cause and Cure*,
"The peculiarity about our modern conception of health is
that it seems to be a purely negative one. So impressed are we
by the myriad presence of disease—so numerous its dangers, so
sudden and unforetellable its attacks—that we have come to
look upon health as the mere absence of the same."

As we continue to eat and live in harmony with nature and
our inner being, we begin to discover new, more vibrant dimensions of life and health. We come to realize that health is
the state of actively harmonizing with our environment, of enjoying life with many other people, and of being able to realize our dreams and ambitions throughout life. When we are
healthy, we meet the following seven conditions:

Freedom from Fatigue

In day-to-day life, we should not feel any fatigue if we are
healthy. After a day's work, we should not complain, "I am
tired." Whatever hardship we may encounter, we should be
able to adapt to it with an energetic desire to work it out har-
moniously. From time to time, we may feel exhausted from
our work, but we should recover after a short rest or night's
sleep. We should not feel mentally tired either. If we frequently change our mind, including our ideas and plans, our
occupation and address, our partner and friends, we are in an
unhealthy state. We lack the vitality to persevere with our
goals and plans, preferring to discard them when difficulties
arise. Under any circumstances, at any time, we should maintain a state of physical and mental balance that is stable, yet
flexible enough to respond immediately to changing circumstances. We will then be able to approach the new environment with a spirit of adventure.

Good Appetite

Throughout our life, each and every day, we should always
have a good appetite for whatever we may encounter: appetite

for food, appetite for sex, appetite for activity, appetite for knowledge, appetite for work, appetite for experience, and appetite for health, freedom, and happiness. Endless appetite is a manifestation of health, and limited appetite is a manifestation of sickness. The bigger our appetite, the richer our life. Without appetite, there is no progress, no development, and no enjoyment. However, in order to keep a large appetite, we should avoid overindulgence. When we are hungry, we should eat so as to satisfy only 80 percent of our hunger, leaving a portion of the stomach unfilled. Satiety reduces our appetite and gradually slows down our metabolism, thinking, activity, and thirst for life. Therefore, we should keep ourselves always hungry, and, as soon as we take in, we should distribute whatever we have received. Keeping emptiness within ourselves is the secret to developing an endless appreciation for life.

Good Sleep

Good sleep is not sleeping for a long time but sleeping soundly for a short time. Good sleep is the result of energetic activity—physical and mental—during the time we are awake. While we are sleeping, we should usually not dream. If we remember a dream after we are awake, it is because our sleep is not deep enough. Nightmares, cloudy dreams, and fragmented dreams are all signs of physical and mental unrest. To see these dreams frequently is a sign of developing mental illness. Suppose we are frequently frightened with the horrors of nightmares. Soon, the precipitating physical and mental qualities will cause "daymares"; awake, we will surround ourselves with groundless suspicions, illusory enemies, and other delusions that turn our life into a battlefield. If we eat macrobiotically and develop our health, we will never suffer such rootless dreams—day or night—of any kind.

Good Memory

Memory is the mother of our judgment. Without memory of what we have experienced, we would have no judgment or ability to evaluate changing circumstances. Good spiritual memory is the foundation of all sound mental activities; they all come out of memory and return to memory. There are various kinds of memory: mechanical memory, such as the remembrance of names and numbers; memory of images, such as the remembrance of scenery and events; and spiritual memory, such as remembrance of where we have come from and how we have realized ourselves in this world at this time. Among these varieties of memory, the most important is the last. It is the memory of spiritual destiny by which we can understand the significance of our lives, know the meaning of the present, and develop an endless appreciation of the past and a limitless aspiration for the future. Good spiritual memory is essential to a meaningful life. All other memories, including mechanical memory and memory of images, are actually part of this memory of our spiritual origin and destiny. As we continue to live macrobiotically, we begin to recover not only memory of past occurrences and present daily events, but also memory of our spiritual destiny. This is one reason why people who share the same food understand each other better.

As our health improves, we find that it is very easy to understand, agree with, and work with other people who are eating the same way, even though they may have been born in different places, brought up and educated in different ways. The reason they can understand each other is that they share a common, universal memory of infinite oneness, whether or not they are aware of it.

Freedom from Anger

If we are in good health, throughout our lifetimes we should never be angry; we are living within the infinite universe and we are all living in harmony with our environment so there is no reason to be angry. We know that everyone, everything, and every phenomenon — including difficulties, sicknesses, and enemies — are complementary to one another. Being angry shows our limitation, our inability to understand and embrace, our lack of patience and perseverance. In Far Eastern countries, the ideograph for anger describes anger as the mind of a slave. Another word for anger means acute sickness in the liver. In Oriental medicine, anger is correlated with liver malfunction, as other major mental and emotional reactions are correlated to disorders of other major organs. Those who do not know how to cope with changing circumstances often become very excited, while those who know how to adapt do not feel any anger. Health is the capacity to accept all circumstances with a smile, change difficulties into opportunities, and turn enemies into friends.

Joyful Responsiveness

In order to live an active and productive life, it is necessary to respond immediately to the constantly changing environment. Life is a continuous progression of such responses. We should be accurate in our expression, swift in our motion, orderly in our behavior, and clear in our thinking. Moment-to-moment responses such as these should be full of joy and humor. Our countenance should be bright, cheerful, and optimistic, and merry thoughts should radiate to everyone around us. Greetings should be exchanged actively with everyone we meet. Like the sun that radiates its light and warmth to everyone, our presence should give joy and happiness to all. Joyousness is a natural result of good health and eating well day to day.

Endless Appreciation

As manifestations of the infinite universe, we should know that all people and all beings are brothers and sisters, accompanying one another on the endless journey of life. We should clearly understand that there is nothing really opposing us. We should clearly know that if we experience difficulties, it is because of some underlying lack of harmony in our way of life; however, this discord can be changed and transformed into its opposite, peacefully, without any conflict or suffering. When we are healthy, we become endlessly appreciative of the universe and all its manifestations. We are healthy when we are able to receive and embrace everything gratefully and when, without hesitation, we are able to give of ourselves — our ideals, our materials, our activity, our energy, and even our life itself—to all from whom and from which we have received. Even when we are physically sick, we are healthy if we are aware that we are the cause of our own sickness, are thankful for the opportunity to learn, and surrender our destiny to nature in a spirit of endless appreciation. Conversely, we may be without any physical or mental symptoms of disease, but unless a deep gratitude permeates our whole life, we are not truly healthy and whole.

ONE GRAIN, TEN THOUSAND GRAINS

The traditional expression, "one grain, ten thousand grains," symbolizes the fact that the Earth returns many grains for every one that it receives. In macrobiotics we use this expression to convey the spirit of helping others by distributing the key to life and health.

Our modern world is in crisis. Practically every family is now suffering from either cancer, heart disease, mental disorders, AIDS, or immune deficiencies. Now more than ever, the world needs the message of hope and recovery that is macrobiotics.

We should all realize that cancer is not solely the concern of cancer patients, their families, or the medical profession. Cancer is merely one dramatic symptom, out of many, of the misconceptions and unbalanced patterns of living that characterize modern life. In a sense, we all have cancer and will continue to be affected by the disease until a new, peaceful way of life is established in place of the old. Cancer is a metaphor for the self-destructive tendencies of modern civilization as a whole. If we can learn to recover from cancer naturally, we may discover that a solution to the multiple ills of society itself is at last on the horizon.

Recommended Reading

Aihara, Herman, *Basic Macrobiotics*. Tokyo & New York: Japan Publications, Inc., 1985.

Benedict, Dirk. *Confessions of a Kamikaze Cowboy*. Garden City Park, N.Y.: Avery Publishing Group, 1991.

Brown, Virginia, with Susan Stayman. *Macrobiotic Miracle: How A Vermont Family Overcame Cancer*. Tokyo & New York: Japan Publications, Inc., 1985.

Dietary Goals for the United States. Washington, D.C.: Select Committee on Nutrition and Human Needs, U.S. Senate, 1977.

Diet, Nutrition and Cancer. Washington, D.C.: National Academy of Sciences, 1982.

Dufty, William. *Sugar Blues*. New York: Warner Books, 1975.

Esko, Edward and Wendy Esko. *Macrobiotic Cooking for Everyone*. Tokyo & New York: Japan Publications, Inc., 1980.

Esko, Wendy. *Aveline Kushi's Introducing Macrobiotic Cooking*. Tokyo and New York: Japan Publications, Inc., 1987.

Fukuoka, Masanobu. *The Natural Way of Farming*. Tokyo & New York: Japan Publications, Inc., 1985.

————. *The One-Straw Revolution*. Emmaus, Pa.: Rodale Press, 1978.

Healthy People: The Surgeon General's Report on Health Promotion and Disease Prevention. Washington, D.C.: Government Printing Office, 1979.

Hiedenry, Carolyn. *Making the Transition to a Macrobiotic Diet*. Garden City Park, N.Y.: Avery Publishing Group, 1987.

Hippocrates. *Hippocratic Writings*. Edited by G. E. R. Lloyd. Translated by J. Chadwick and W. N. Mann. New York: Penguin Books, 1978.

Ineson, John. *The Way of Life: Macrobiotics and the Spirit of Christianity*. Tokyo & New York: Japan Publications, Inc., 1986.

Jacobs, Leonard and Barbara Leonard. *Cooking with Seitan*. Tokyo & New York: Japan Publications, Inc., 1986.

Jacobson, Michael. *The Changing American Diet*. Washington, D.C.: Center for Science in the Public Interest, 1978.

Kaibara, Ekiken. *Yojokun: Japanese Secrets of Good Health*. Tokyo: Tokuma Shoten, 1974.

Kohler, Jean and Mary Alice. *Healing Miracles from Macrobiotics*. West Nyack, N.Y.: Parker, 1979.

Kotsch, Ronald. *Macrobiotics: Yesterday and Today*. Tokyo & New York: Japan Publications, Inc., 1985.

Kushi, Aveline. *How to Cook with Miso*. Tokyo & New York: Japan Publications, Inc., 1978.

————. *Lessons of Night and Day*. Garden City Park, N.Y.: Avery Publishing Group, 1985.

————. *Macrobiotic Food and Cooking Series: Diabetes and Hypoglycemia; Allergies*. Tokyo & New York: Japan Publications, Inc., 1985.

————. *Macrobiotic Food and Cooking Series: Obesity, Weight Loss, and Eating Disorders; Infertility and Reproductive Disorders*. Tokyo & New York: Japan Publications, Inc., 1987.

Kushi, Aveline, with Alex Jack. *Aveline Kushi's Complete Guide to Macrobiotic Cooking*. New York: Warner Books, 1985.

Kushi, Aveline and Michio Kushi. *Macrobiotic Pregnancy and Care of the Newborn*. Edited by Edward and Wendy Esko. Tokyo & New York: Japan Publications, Inc., 1984.

_____. *Macrobiotic Child Care and Family Health*. Tokyo & New York: Japan Publications, Inc., 1986.

Kushi, Aveline and Wendy Esko. *Aveline Kushi's Introducing Macrobiotic Cooking*. Tokyo & New York: Japan Publications, 1987.

_____. *Aveline Kushi's Wonderful World of Salads*. Tokyo & New York: Japan Publications, 1989.

_____. *The Changing Seasons Macrobiotic Cookbook*. Garden City Park, N.Y.: Avery Publishing Group, 1985.

_____. *The Good Morning Macrobiotic Breakfast Book*. Garden City Park, N.Y.: Avery Publishing Group, 1991.

_____. *The Macrobiotic Cancer Prevention Cookbook*. Garden City Park, N.Y.: Avery Publishing Group, 1988.

_____. *Macrobiotic Family Favorites*. Tokyo & New York: Japan Publications, Inc., 1987.

_____. *The New Pasta Cuisine: Low-Fat Noodle and Pasta Dishes From Around the World*. Tokyo & New York: Japan Publications, 1991.

_____. *The Quick and Natural Macrobiotic Cookbook*. Chicago, Ill.: Contemporary Books, 1989.

Kushi, Michio, *The Book of Dō-In: Exercise for Physical and Spiritual Development*. Tokyo & New York: Japan Publications, Inc. 1979.

_____. *The Book of Macrobiotics: The Universal Way of Health, Happiness and Peace*. Tokyo & New York: Japan Publications, Inc., 1986 (Rev. ed).

_____. *Cancer and Heart Disease: The Macrobiotic Approach to Degenerative Disorders*. Tokyo & New York: Japan Publications, Inc., 1986 (Rev. ed).

_____. *Crime and Diet: The Macrobiotic Approach*. Tokyo & New York: Japan Publications, Inc., 1987.

_____. *The Era of Humanity*. Brookline, Mass.: East West Journal, 1980.

_____. *How to See Your Health: The Book of Oriental Diagnosis*. Tokyo & New York: Japan Publications, Inc., 1980.

_____. *Macrobiotic Health Education Series: Diabetes and Hypoglycemia; Allergies*. Tokyo & New York: Japan Publications, Inc., 1985.

_____. *Macrobiotic Health Education Series: Obesity, Weight Loss, and Eating Disorders; Infertility and Repro-*

ductive Disorders. Tokyo & New York: Japan Publications, Inc., 1987.

_____. *Natural Healing through Macrobiotics*. Tokyo & New York: Japan Publications, Inc. 1987.

_____. *On the Greater View: Collected Thoughts on Macrobiotics and Humanity*. Garden City Park, N.Y.: Avery Publishing Group, 1985.

_____. *Your Face Never Lies*. Garden City Park, N.Y.: Avery Publishing Group, 1983.

Kushi, Michio and Alex Jack. *The Cancer Prevention Diet*. New York: St. Martin's Press, 1983.

_____. *Diet for a Strong Heart*. New York: St. Martin's Press, 1984.

Kushi, Michio, with Alex Jack. *One Peaceful World*. New York: St. Martin's Press, 1987.

Kushi, Michio, with Edward and Wendy Esko. *Gentle Art of Making Love, The*. Garden City Park, N.Y.: Avery Publishing Group, 1990.

Kushi, Michio and Aveline Kushi, with Alex Jack. *The Macrobiotic Diet*. Tokyo & New York: Japan Publications, Inc., 1985.

Kushi, Michio, with Stephen Blauer. *The Macrobiotic Way*. Garden City Park, N.Y.: Avery Publishing Group, 1985.

Lerman, Andrea Bliss. *Macrobiotic Community Cookbook, The*. Garden City Park, N.Y.: Avery Publishing Group, 1989.

Mendelsohn, Robert S., M.D. *Confessions of a Medical Heretic*. Chicago: Contemporary Books, 1979.

_____. *Male Practice*. Chicago: Contemporary Books, 1980.

Nussbaum, Elaine. *Recovery: From Cancer to Health through Macrobiotics*. Tokyo & New York: Japan Publications, Inc. 1986.

Nutrition and Mental Health. Washington, D.C.: Select Committee on Nutrition and Human Needs, U.S. Senate, 1977, 1980.

Ohsawa, George. *Cancer and the Philosophy of the Far East*. Oroville, Calif.: George Ohsawa Macrobiotic Foundation, 1971 edition.

_____. *You Are All Sanpaku*. Edited by William Dufty. New York: University Books, 1965.

_____. *Zen Macrobiotics*. Los Angeles: Ohsawa Foundation, 1965.

Price, Western, A., D.D.S. *Nutrition and Physical Degeneration*. Santa Monica, Calif.: Price-Pottenger Nutritional Foundation, 1945.

Sattilaro, Anthony, M.D., with Tom Monte. *Recalled by Life: The Story of My Recovery from Cancer*. Boston: Houghton-Mifflin, 1982.

Scott, Neil E., with Jean Farmer. *Eating with Angels*. Tokyo & New York: Japan Publications, Inc., 1986.

Tara, William. *Macrobiotics and Human Behavior*. Tokyo & New York: Japan Publications, Inc., 1985.

Yamamoto, Shizuko. *Barefoot Shiatsu*. Tokyo & New York: Japan Publications, Inc., 1979.

The Yellow Emperor's Classic of Internal Medicine. Translated by Ilza Veith, Berkeley: University of California Press, 1979.

Macrobiotic Resources

Macrobiotic Way of Life Seminar

The Macrobiotic Way of Life Seminar is an introductory program offered by the Kushi Institute in Massachusetts. It is a complete guide to beginning macrobiotics and includes classes in macrobiotic cooking, home care, and kitchen setup, lectures on the philosophy of macrobiotics and the standard diet, and individual guidance in adopting a new way of life. The seminar is presented monthly by Michio Kushi and associate teachers.

Macrobiotic Residential Seminar

The Macrobiotic Residential Seminar is an introductory program offered at the Kushi Institute of the Berkshires in western Massachusetts. It is a one-week live-in program that features hands-on training in macrobiotic cooking and home care, lectures on the philosophy and practice of macrobiotics, and meals prepared by a specially trained cooking staff. It is presented twice per month.

Other Programs

The Kushi Institute offers a variety of introductory, intermediate, and advanced level programs on all aspects of macrobiotics, in Becket and in cities throughout North America. Special programs include an annual Macrobiotic Summer Conference with participants from around the world, and ongoing seminars by Michio Kushi on topics such as macrobiotic health care, spiritual development, and philosophy. For information on any of these programs, contact:

Kushi Institute of the Berkshires
Box 7
Becket, Massachusetts 01223
(413) 623-5742

One Peaceful World

One Peaceful World is an international information network and friendship society of macrobiotic friends, families, educational centers, organic farmers, traditional food producers, teachers and parents, authors and artists, publishers and business people, and other individuals and organizations around the world devoted to the realization of one healthy, peaceful world. Activities include educational and spiritual tours, assemblies and forums, international food and agricultural projects, the One Peaceful World Village and Children's Memorial and Shrine in Becket, the quarterly *One Peaceful World Newsletter*, and other communications.

For membership information and a current catalog of publications and videos, contact:

One Peaceful World
Box 10
Becket, Massachusetts 01223
(413) 623-5742

About the Authors

Michio Kushi, the leader of the international macrobiotic community, was born in Japan and studied international law and political science at Tokyo University. He came to the United States in 1949 and is the founder and chairman of the Kushi Institute, the Kushi Foundation, and One Peaceful World. He has given seminars on Oriental medicine and philosophy at the United Nations and served as advisor to governments in Europe, Africa, and Latin America. He is the author of several dozen books including *The Cancer Prevention Diet*, *The Book of Macrobiotics*, *The Macrobiotic Way*, and *One Peaceful World*, and lives in Becket and Brookline, Massachusetts with his wife, Aveline, also a leading voice in macrobiotic education.

Edward Esko helped pioneer macrobiotic education in North America in the 1970s and '80s. He began studies with Michio Kushi in 1971 and has taught macrobiotic philosophy and health care throughout the United States and in Europe, South America, and Japan. He is on the faculty of the Kushi Institute of the Berkshires, and has co-authored or edited several popular books including *Natural Healing through Macrobiotics*, *Doctors Look at Macrobiotics*, and *Macrobiotic Child Care and Family Health*. He lives with his wife, Wendy, and seven children in Becket, Massachusetts.

Index

Agriculture, 13, 14, 26, 28, 29
AIDS, 9, 41
Allergies, 20, 48
American Cancer Society, 67, 72-74, 120
American Diabetes Association, 66
American Heart Association, 66
American Medical Association, 65, 74, 77
American Society for Clinical Nutrition, 66
Anatomy, human, 24-25
Anemia, 79
Anger, 158-159
Animal foods, 102-103, 103-105, 108, 115
Antibodies, 21
Anti-insulin, 61
Appetite, 156-157
Appreciation, 159-160

Ascorbic acid. *See* Vitamins, C.
Awareness, 16

Beans, 36, 39, 103, 105-107, 129-130
Benedict, Dirk, 2
Beta-Cartone, 118, 122, 128. *See also* Vitamins, A.
Beverages, 30, 37, 144-145. *See also* water.
Biopsies, numbers of, 10
Bladder. *See* cancer, bladder.
Blampied, Doug. *See* case histories.
Blood, cleansing of, 43
Blood pressure, 2, 92
Body scrubbing, 42
Bone marrow harvest, 32
Bone marrow transplant, 32
Bowel motility, 42, 43
Brain tumor, 11, 150-154